Kick-start Your Plant-Based Lifestyle 2-in-1 Bundle

Plant-Based Diet is the Solution + Plant-Based Diet Cookbook – The #1 Beginners Guide for Ultimate Nutrition, Complete With Meal Plan

By: Alyani Cook

Kick-start Your Plant-Based Lifestyle

Kick-start Your Plant-Based Lifestyle

Copyright © 2019 - All rights reserved.

This document is geared towards providing exact and reliable information in regards to the topic and issue covered. The publication is sold with the idea that the publisher is not required to render accounting, officially permitted, or otherwise, qualified services. If advice is necessary, legal or professional, a practiced individual in the profession should be ordered.

From a Declaration of Principles which was accepted and approved equally by a Committee of the American Bar Association and a Committee of Publishers and Associations.

In no way is it legal to reproduce, duplicate, or transmit any part of this document in either electronic means or in printed format. Recording of this publication is strictly prohibited and any storage of this document is not allowed unless with written permission from the publisher. All rights reserved.

The information provided herein is stated to be truthful and consistent, in that any liability, in terms of inattention or otherwise, by any usage or abuse of any policies, processes, or directions contained within is the solitary and utter responsibility of the recipient reader. Under no circumstances will any legal responsibility or blame be held against the publisher for any reparation, damages, or monetary loss due to the information herein, either directly or indirectly.

Respective authors own all copyrights not held by the publisher.

The information herein is offered for informational purposes solely, and is universal as so. The presentation of the information is without contract or any type of guarantee assurance.

The trademarks that are used are without any consent, and the publication of the trademark is without permission or backing by the trademark owner. All trademarks and brands within this book are for clarifying purposes only and are the owned by the owners themselves, not affiliated with this document.

Kick-start Your Plant-Based Lifestyle

Kick-start Your Plant-Based Lifestyle

TABLE OF CONTENTS

Introduction	10
Chapter 1: What is a Plant-based Diet?	14
Chapter 2: Benefits of a Plant-based Diet	29
Chapter 3: Common Misconceptions About the Plant-based Diet	52
Chapter 4: Who is the Plant-based Diet for?	68
Chapter 5: Foods to Enjoy and Avoid on a Plant-based Diet	83
Chapter 6: Grocery List and Meal Plan	101
Chapter 7: Tips and Tricks for Real Life	139
Chapter 8: The Secret to Success	149
Conclusion	160

Kick-start Your Plant-Based Lifestyle

Plant-Based Diet Cookbook Foreword	165
What is a Plant-based Diet?	166
In The Spring	172
In The Summer	180
In The Fall	191
In The Winter	201
Last Words	214

Kick-start Your Plant-Based Lifestyle

Your Free Gift!

As a way of showing my sincere gratitude for your purchase, I'm offering a *FREE* complementary download for **17 Meal Plan Templates** that is *EXCLUSIVE* to readers of *"Kick-start Your Plant-Based Lifestyle 2-in-1 Bundle"* only.

These 17 Meal Plan Templates are not only *beautifully* designed, they are also practical tools that will help you stay on track on your Plant-based Diet. Because as you'll learn later in this book, meal planning is key to staying on a diet.

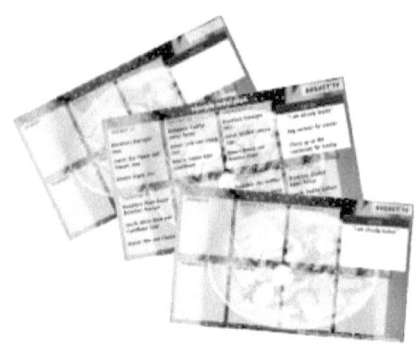

Simply type in

>><http://tiny.cc/mdl1az> <<

to get Your Free Gift today.

Plant-based Diet is the Solution – A Beginner's Guidebook

How To Get Nutrition, Own A Healthy Lifestyle While Saving The World

By: Alyani Cook

Introduction

We're only given one planet to live on. It's here on earth that we create our lives, share memories with loved ones, and try to make them all count. My name is Alyani Cook, and I am a mother of two beautiful boys. Much like every other mother out there, my dream is to create a lifestyle where I can be healthy and save the planet along the way so my boys can enjoy it when I'm gone.

I used to be severely overweight and riddled with health problems. One day, while I was researching on different diets to help with my health conditions, I stumbled upon the plant-based diet. At first, it seemed too good to be true. A diet that was able to lower my cholesterol, help me lose weight, and benefit the planet?

Sure enough, I found studies after studies that support how a whole food, plant-based diet could improve my health conditions. In addition, it is also a wonderful diet to not only change my health but also the world I wish for my boys to grow up in.

As you probably could have guessed by now, a plant-based diet is a diet that consists of foods that derive from plants. These foods range from vegetables to grains and even fruits. While many individuals refer to this diet as a vegan or vegetarian diet, it is so much more than that. While some choose to eat a small amount of meat, I will show you the secrets and benefits a plant-based diet can bring you.

At this point in time, there are about four billion individuals who follow a plant-based diet. One of my favorite aspects of the plant-based diet is all of the research placed behind the facts to support the evidence. One of the top gurus of the plant-based diet is Dr. Campbell who is a professor at Cornell University. He alone has spent a few decades learning the incredible health and nutritional benefits a plant-based diet can bring. He is also the co-author of a book known as "The China Study", where he spent about 2 decades researching the diet in China to help others fight disease through diet. In fact, he was the first one to coin the term, "whole food, plant-based."

Other gurus who have researched and studied the plant-based diet include Dr. McDougall, Dr. Esselstyn, Dr. Barnard and more! Each doctor has done his own research and found how beneficial a plant-based diet can be. If you are ready to change your life, improve your health, and save the planet, this diet is perfect for you!

In the next few chapters, we will be going over everything you need to know to help you get started on the plant-based diet. As I've mentioned earlier, I only happened to stumble upon this diet, but I was so impressed by it that I got hooked onto studying about it. Now that I've done most of the research out there, I've decided to compile them all into this one book, so you have one ultimate source to refer to and be set up for absolute success. Honestly, this diet and lifestyle has changed my life and became so much bigger than myself; I am confident that it can change yours too if you're willing to put in the work.

If you're like me and you've selected this book, then I know you are all about your health and our planet. By making a few changes to your diet, I'm sure we can accomplish this together!

I am so excited to dive right into it and share my

knowledge with you. I sincerely hope that this book will give you a wealth of insights and value.

So before we get started, I would appreciate it if you could do me a simple favor. That is once you're done with this book, please leave me a quick review on Amazon.com.

Thank you!

Chapter One:
What is a Plant-based Diet?

One of the first questions I asked myself when I stumbled upon the plant-based diet was, "how is this diet going to be any different from the rest?" It is an important question as there are so many different diets on the market nowadays. Each diet claims to save your life, get rid of your disease and help you lose weight. At the end of the day, although not every diet is for everyone, you can never go wrong with being more conscious of what you eat.

The plant-based diet puts an emphasis on eating both fresh and whole ingredients. Basically, you are going to want to avoid food that has been highly processed. By eating minimally processed foods and increasing the plants in your diet, it will be effective in helping you to lose weight, improve your health, or both!

Kick-start Your Plant-Based Lifestyle

While there is no true definition to a plant-based diet, it is so much more than a diet. Most diets set you up for failure. If you're anything like me, you must have tried a handful of them already. Many individuals follow strict rules like cutting sugar, cutting carbs, or completely eliminating food groups that they love. Unfortunately, it's hard to do it this way because it's hard to just drop your bad habits. On the other hand, a plant-based diet doesn't have strict rules like these. Instead, it has basic principles that anyone can follow on their own time and pace. The best part is that it is inclusive, so you can make this lifestyle a family event!

Often times, a plant-based diet is confused with a vegan or vegetarian diet. While they are very similar, they are not exactly the same. The best way to describe it is that a plant-based diet is the umbrella term where veganism and vegetarianism falls under. A plant-based diet is extremely versatile to help fit the needs of a variety of people. Yes, there is an emphasis on whole foods that have been minimally processed, but technically, animal products are still allowed on this diet, though they should be limited!

Instead of focusing on the foods that you can't have, you'll be encouraged to learn how to enjoy new types of food such as nuts, seeds, legumes, whole grains, fruits, and vegetables. Later in the chapters of this book, you'll even be provided with a grocery list, meal plan, and the foods you should avoid and the foods you should enjoy. As I said, I'm setting you up for complete success here! When we do this together, we'll also be able to save our planet one healthy person at a time.

Of course, thinking about moving to this diet is going to be your first step. While it sounds like an excellent idea, often times it is difficult to know where to start. The next few chapters will introduce you to the incredible benefits of the diet, who it is for, and some tips and tricks to help you get started.

What is Whole-Food, Plant-Based?

Unfortunately, a plant-based diet is often thought of as boring and bland. While for some people, avoiding animal ingredients is incredibly limiting, you'll soon find out that as you become more innovative with your cooking skills, you will learn to create new flavors. As you try out some of the recipes provided in chapter 6, you'll discover flavors you did not know were even possible.

In order to understand the diet, it's important that you first understand its definition. When I say whole food, it simply refers to foods that are in their natural state. This means that the foods included on this diet are minimally refined, unrefined, or whole and raw.

As for the word "plant-based", this just means the bulk or base of your meal is primarily coming from plants. However, when I say "plant-based foods", this means the food comes directly from plant sources. We will be going over in greater detail in the next section but all you need to know at this point is that plant-based foods do not contain any animal products like honey, eggs, milk or meat. If you're thinking to yourself, that's a majority of my diet; don't worry, you are not alone! That's because you've been brought up on S.A.D, also known as the Standard American Diet, which is the diet of most Americans. While switching to a plant-based diet may take some extra work, it is absolutely worth it because you're doing it for your health and for the health of the environment.

What Are Plant Foods?

You will see me refer to "plant foods" many times throughout this book. When I say, "plant food," I simply mean food that isn't from an animal in any shape or form. Some of the foods include potatoes, fruits, vegetables, legumes, mushrooms and more.

One type of foods that are often confused with

plant foods is plant fragments. Plant fragments are refined foods including chips, oil, sugar, and all-purpose flour. While these foods technically come from plants and do not contain any animal products, they are not considered plant foods. Plant foods must be whole or minimally processed.

You might be scratching your head at this point; I will clarify with an example. An apple is considered a plant food. An apple pie is not a plant food, nor is it plant-based. That is because typically, pies are prepared with milk and eggs. Another example is frozen corn. Frozen corn is considered a plant food while high fructose corn syrup is not because the syrup contains a high amount of processed sugar. Get the picture?

What Does Plant-based Mean?

If someone tells you that they follow a plant-based diet, this means that their diet consists mainly of plant foods. Unless you are told otherwise, you can assume that this individual avoids animal-based products like gelatin, butter, milk, eggs, and animal meat, or they eat them very minimally. These individuals will also avoid eating plant fragments and place their focus on whole plant foods instead.

Kick-start Your Plant-Based Lifestyle

There will be a learning curve if you're just starting this diet but that does not mean it is impossible. You'd even be surprised to learn which foods are plant-based and which are not. While you may need to give up some of your favorite treats, I assure you there are some delicious alternatives out there. One of my favorite aspects of a plant-based diet is that you won't have to count calories. In fact, your diet will be filled to the brim with so much nutrient-dense foods that you'll never go hungry again, provided you're following the diet the correct way.

Minimally Processed Plant-based Foods

I know, a lot of new terms are being thrown at you right now. Although it is a lot to take in at first, keep holding on. You will soon be a plant-based expert! It is vital that you understand all of these terms before diving into the diet so that you are well prepared for success. Knowledge truly is a powerful concept when it comes to succeeding with anything in life.

While you may think you understand what minimally processed means, you may be surprised to find that certain foods are more processed than you thought. Some examples are granola bars, corn tortillas, and breakfast cereals. While they are technically accepted as plant-based, they are actually highly processed. Just check out their labels and you'll see.

Some foods that are more minimally processed include oatmeal, peanut butter, salsa, applesauce, hummus, and even guacamole. Condiments like vinegar, soy sauce, hot sauce, and mustard are also considered minimally processed.

Two food items that cause a bit of confusion are mushrooms and yeast. While they are not technically considered plants, I believe they can be consumed on a plant-based diet.

Another food that is often questioned is bread. While bread is suitable for most plant-based eaters, you will need to read its nutrient label to make a better judgment. Some breads that are sold commercially could potentially contain stabilizers, fillers, eggs and dairy. Obviously, this would mean that the bread is no longer fully plant-based. Luckily, there are many different types of breads out there for you to try that are still within the guidelines of your diet.

Plant-based Diet Reference

As the plant-based diet grows in popularity and is being introduced to a wider audience, some people have modified and created different versions of it in order to fit their needs. The following diets are the most common ones.

- Veganism

Veganism is a diet that includes only seeds, nuts, grains, legumes, and vegetables. Often times, you will hear vegan and plant-based being used interchangeably. Later, we will be going over why they are not necessarily the same thing. However, in a nutshell, veganism is a lifestyle choice where an individual chooses to have no animal sources in their life from clothing to food choices.

There are two main categories of veganism at this point in time. First, you have fruitarianism; this is a diet that consists primarily of fruit. The second is raw veganism. A raw vegan will eat foods that are uncooked or dehydrated. Obviously, both of these are very restrictive for a beginner, which is not what a plant-based diet should be.

- Vegetarianism

A vegetarian will eat foods such as seeds, nuts, fruits, legumes, and vegetables, much like a vegan. They are similar in that they both do not eat meat. The main difference between a vegetarian and a vegan is that vegetarians still include eggs and dairy in their diet. There are several types of vegetarianism including ovo-lacto; includes dairy and eggs, ovo; includes eggs but no dairy, and lacto; which includes dairy but no eggs. You also have semi-vegetarians who eat mostly a vegetarian diet but will have meat on special occasions.

Another version of the vegetarian diet is the macrobiotic diet. This diet consists of naturally processed foods, sea vegetables, beans, vegetables, and whole grains.

- Pescetarianism

There is also a pescatarian who follows a semi-vegetarian diet, but includes seafood, dairy, and eggs.

As you can see, there are many different alternatives. Although a plant-based diet is not an easy change if you've had the average American diet for the longest time, its flexibility makes it perfectly do-able. As I've stated earlier, you are being provided with all of the information you need in one book to help get you started! At the end of the day, the responsibility still rests on your shoulders to put in the work and tailor your diet according to your needs and desires.

Plant-based Benefits for the Environment

In the next chapter, you will be learning all the incredible health benefits the plant-based diet can bring you, but it is so much bigger than that. When you switch your lifestyle to being plant-based, you are also helping to

Kick-start Your Plant-Based Lifestyle

save the environment. At the end of the day, what better gift can you give your children and loved ones than a cleaner and more beautiful environment to prosper in? With so much destruction in the world today, why not do your part?

For those of us who love our planet, it is a very scary world out there! Animal and plant habitats alike are being destroyed by deforestation. On top of that, we're facing global warming. By switching to a plant-based diet, you will be cutting down your carbon footprint and helping to protect the earth for future generations to come. You would be amazed to learn how much the animal-based industry of agriculture adds to our poor earth's woes. In fact, the factory farms in the United States produce about 300 million tons of waste every year! On top of that, these farms are also polluting our air and making us sicker than ever before. If you care about the environment, there are several ways a plant-based diet can help.

Cut Your Carbon Footprint

As of right now, the United Nations Food and Agriculture Organization has estimated that the production of livestock is responsible for a whopping 14.5% of global greenhouse gas emissions. It is believed that just cattle alone, which are raised for beef and milk, are responsible for 65% of these emissions. The other sources of these emissions come from the feed processing and production to keep these animals alive.

As mentioned earlier, these animals produce about 300 million tons of waste per year. This waste is responsible for 37% of the agricultural greenhouse gas emissions. It is believed that there is a management factory farm referred to as lagoons where there are cesspits filled to the brim with this animal waste. This waste produces large quantities of methane, which is responsible for warming the earth about 20 times faster than carbon dioxide.

By switching over to a plant-based diet, you are massively decreasing or even totally cutting out animal products from your diet. In other words, you are reducing your carbon footprint by not contributing to this industry. While it may not seem like much, if everyone plays his or her individual part, it can make a significant difference.

Start Conserving Water

For most diets, it isn't specified clearly what beverages are recommended. Well, on the plant-based diet, a beverage you should be cutting down on will be milk. According to the Water Footprint Network, they have estimated that it takes around 1000 gallons of water in order to produce 1 gallon of milk. Also, it takes up to 6 times more water to produce 1 pound of animal protein compared to 1 pound of grain protein. More water is also needed for animal produce versus plant produce. The Twente Water Centre from the University of Twente has calculated that beef uses approximately 20 times more water than grains or potatoes.

When you go on a plant-based diet, you'd be reducing consumption of animal-products and thus, help to reduce the amount of water being used. You see, water is a very precious resource. What would happen if our children have to live in a world with no fresh water? That is why we need to pave the road towards a healthier planet today, for the sake of our future generations. At this point, it is no longer just about you or me. We must do what is best for the future of the entire human race.

Cleaner Air

Clean air is incredibly important. This is a resource that we all need in order to survive. Humans need it; animals need it, planet earth needs it. The manure from livestock is producing a potent form of nitrogen, more commonly referred to as ammonia. This ammonia is killing off algae, fish, and even adds smog into our cities. Studies have also found that the air surrounding factory farms have above-average levels of carbon dioxide, endotoxins, and hydrogen sulfide, and all of these are terrible for our environment. Again, switching to a plant-based diet means that you'll be helping to alleviate all these toxins from our planet.

Love Animals, Don't Eat Them!

One of the major reasons people succeed in switching to veganism or vegetarianism is due to their deep love for animals. If you are like me and you can't stand the thought of eating a living being that has some form of intelligence and sentience, then cutting animal protein out of your diet should be pretty easy. That's not all. On top of saving the animals, you'll also be helping to save the habitats of these animals. Animal agriculture is a huge contributor to desertification and deforestation of our planet. Studies have shown that animal agriculture takes about one-third of the arable land in the world. By taking up and damaging so much natural land, we could eventually see the extinction of many animal species such as sloths, red pandas, and orangutans.

The Power of Plant-based

Kick-start Your Plant-Based Lifestyle

While the animal agriculture does make up the core of our environmental issues, there are other factors leading to global warming and greenhouse gas emissions too. Similarly, there are several other contributing factors to land degradation, deforestation, and extinction. While it all does seem rather bleak, make no mistake that you still have the power to make a difference.

Two of the biggest problems we face today are global warming and eating ourselves to more diseases and even our deaths. However, the real problem is that most people are unwilling to do anything about it. What many people do not know is that we have the ability to fight against climate change, and it happens to start right on our plates. By making proper food choices, we are taking back control of our own survival, all while creating true sustainability for future generations to come.

While we may be unable to change the future of our world overnight, we cannot underestimate the power of everyday habits. By choosing one plant-based meal today, it increases the odds of you choosing a plant-based meal tomorrow and then another plant-based meal the day after. As you begin to eat healthier, you're contributing to the demand and supply for plant produce. This ensures that vital crop resources are being prioritized to feed human beings as opposed to livestock. It also lets farmers know that plant produce is in-demand and a lucrative alternative to animal produce. The more people switch to a plant-based diet, the more available plant-based options will be made for us. As individuals come together, I believe we truly will be able to make a difference in this world.

Of course, these are long-term benefits. However, a plant-based diet can also benefit your personal life right now. In the next chapter, you'll be learning just how efficiently whole foods can change your life for the better. From weight loss to improving your health conditions, a plant-based diet can change your life in ways you never even expected.

Chapter Two:
Benefits of a Plant-based Diet

While saving the planet is an added bonus, this diet will be able to benefit your personal health and overall well-being in so many different ways. Whether you are looking to improve your health, lose weight or combat certain illnesses, the plant-based diet can surely bring a positive change for you.

Of course, every diet on the market makes these crazy claims about changing your life. The difference with the plant-based diet is that there is actual science behind these claims and I've extracted as many of them to be used as evidence. Studies after studies have been done on this diet, to prove that it can really benefit you. We will now go over some of the incredible benefits a plant-based diet can bring to your life.

Eczema and Acne

Did you know that more than 85% of adults and teenagers have acne? According to research, scientists believe that there may be a link between hormonal acne and insulin resistance. Due to the Western diet being higher in glycemic index, this often causes insulin resistance. When insulin resistance happens, it changes the sebum production in the body, which is what controls your oil secretions. So when your sebum production gets messed up, it'll then cause inflammation and acne.

In the same study, the researchers also found that there is a possible link between acne and cow's milk. This could be due to the hormones in cow's milk, which has insulin-like growth factors. These hormones in the cow's milk are meant for baby calves, not human babies. So when children are given this milk in the early stages of their life, the milk gives them skin irritations, such as eczema. In fact, 81% of children have such reactions, and the research has shown that eggs and cow's milk were the primary causes.

If you have acne or eczema, it might be your body reacting adversely to eggs or cow's milk. Often times when people begin a plant-based diet, they see a difference instantly. As you begin to increase the fruits, fibers, vegetables, and decrease the dairy in your diet, you will be healing both your skin and your overall health!

Baby Making and Fertility

Fertility is more important to some people compared to others. If you personally experience Polycystic Ovary Syndrome also known as PCOS, imbalanced hormones, or infertility, they could all be due to an insulin resistance in your body. According to studies, if you have animal products in your body, this could potentially predispose you to acidity. With an acidic body, this creates the perfect breeding ground for bacteria. In turn, this could potentially sap your energy and decrease your immunity. If you're trying to become pregnant, this is bad because a weakened immune system puts your body on high alert, essentially harming the sperm and development of embryos. It has also been found that a weakened immune system increases the chances of miscarriages and the contribution to infections.

A study from the American Journal of Obstetrics & Gynecology has shown that 5% of the total energy intake of a vegetable protein compared to an animal protein was linked to a 50% lower risk of ovulatory infertility. This means that if you would just increase the number of plant-based foods in your diet, you could decrease the chances of infertility. If you personally struggle with fertility issues, switching to a plant-based diet could be worth a shot.

Migraine and Stroke Risks

Migraines, unfortunately, affect people in a number of ways. For some, these headaches happen only once or twice a week; for others, it might strike several times a day. The factors that trigger this pain also vary from person to person. The only similarity that can be agreed upon is that migraines cause pain that disrupts your daily life.

In a study on 42 adults who suffered from migraines, the adults were asked to follow a 36-week regiment of a low-fat, plant-based, vegan diet. Each patient in this trial was accessed in the beginning, in the middle, and at the end. By the end, the average frequency of their headaches declined after following the plant-based diet.

Research has also shown that a plant-based diet may help minimize the risk of having a stroke. This could be due to the fact that a plant-based diet is high in fiber, specifically at least 25 grams of soluble fiber and 47 grams of insoluble fiber. In the next chapter, I'll be revealing to you what you can eat, but generally you'll be getting this fiber from delicious foods like whole wheat, brown rice, nuts, oats, and beans!

Reverse Diabetes

You may not know this, but more than 20 million people in the United States have been diagnosed with diabetes. Since 1990, this number has tripled! Unfortunately, around 132,000 children and kids under the age of 18 suffer from diabetes. In 2014 alone, 52,139 people developed end-stage renal disease due to diabetes. Due to such an epidemic, it costs about $245 billion to diagnose diabetes in the United States alone. Unfortunately, according to the National Vital Statistics Reports, diabetes leads to about 750,000 deaths in a single year. That number is way too high when there is a simple solution to the problem. Not only can a plant-based diet prevent diabetes, it can even help to reverse it.

Studies have shown that a plant-based diet can drop your risk of diabetes and hypertension very significantly. This has something to do with insulin resistance, which is the leading cause of type 2 diabetes. Basically, insulin is needed for the glucose in our bloodstream to be absorbed into our cells to produce energy. When there is insulin resistance, glucose cannot get absorbed into our cells and gets piled up in our bloodstream instead. This then leads to health complications. A study from Nutrients journal found that plant-based diet helps to increase our insulin sensitivity. So, now you know that this diet can definitely help prevent diabetes, but more importantly it can also reverse it.

There was a study done on adults who have type 2 diabetes. They were split into 2 groups. The first group was asked to follow a vegan diet that consisted of 10% fat, 15% protein and 75% carbohydrates. The food that they could eat on their specific diet included legumes, grains, fruits, and vegetables. The second group was asked to follow a diet provided by the American Diabetes Association. By the end of the experiment, 43% of the participants from the first group were able to reduce their diabetes medications. This is way more compared to the 26% in the second group, who were following the diet recommended by the American Diabetes Association. In fact, these individuals were able to turn their life around in as little as 22 weeks! On top of that, they also lowered their total cholesterol and LDL cholesterol, also known as "bad" cholesterol, in 74 weeks.

Boosting Your Immune System

Kick-start Your Plant-Based Lifestyle

Our immune system is a very important factor for our health. As a result, scientists began to study how fruits and vegetables intake affects our health. According to a study from The American Journal of Clinical Nutrition, they found that adults who choose to eat 5 or more servings of fruits and vegetables per day had a 93% rise in antibody responses. This is in comparison to adults who eat less than 3 servings of fruits and vegetables per day.

Learning how to fuel your body is important if you're looking to prevent diseases before it has the chance to attack your system. Luckily, there are several immune boosting foods that can be found in a plant-based diet. One of the tastier ones are citrus fruits!

When people fall sick, they often turn to vitamin C. It helps to increase the number of white blood cells in your body and is the key to fighting infections. Some delicious and popular fruits you can try to include in your diet are lemons, limes, tangerines, clementine, oranges, and grapefruit. Getting your vitamin C is important, as our bodies are incapable of producing or storing it. Due to this factor, you will need to consume it daily for continued health.

While citrus foods are believed to have the most vitamin C, you may be surprised to learn that red bell pepper has twice as much! They are also rich in beta carotene, which is in charge of keeping your skin and eyes healthy. Other foods that can help boost your immune system include broccoli, garlic, ginger, spinach, yogurt, almonds, and more! Later in this book, you will be provided with a meal plan and recipes that will include many of these delicious foods.

Breast Cancer Risk Reduction

Breast cancer can be a scary prognosis to receive, but with a plant-based diet, you can greatly reduce your risk of getting it in the first place. Studies have shown that if you limit your alcohol intake, eat foods that are mostly plant-based, and maintain a normal body weight; you could reduce your risk of developing breast cancer by 60%.

A plant-based diet can help in several different aspects of your health. However, scientists were curious as to how cancer relates to the intake of meat. There was actually a study published in the Epidemiology Journal where it was found that individuals who have a diet consisting of low vegetables and high meat intake, had their risk of developing breast cancer raised by 74%!

I look forward to seeing your thoughts! Now let's keep

going.

Kidney Stones

Studies have shown that there's a correspondence between the consumption of animal proteins and the number of discharges for stones. These animal proteins include poultry, fish, and meat. The study showed a link between higher kidney stone incidents and higher meat intake. In fact, some studies have shown that eating just one extra can of tuna in a single day can increase an individual's risk of forming a stone in the urinary tract by 250%! That is a huge jump for just one can of animal protein.

High Blood Pressure and Heart Disease Prevention

As of right now, 1 in 3 Americans has high blood pressure. A specific study published in The American Journal of Clinical Nutrition was done on 545,000 women and men between the ages of 50 to 71 and it has found that as individuals make their diet more plant-based, they were able to reduce their hypertension rates. In fact, simply by switching from an omnivore to a vegan diet caused a 75% drop in hypertension.

The same study was also found that a vegetarian

diet helps protect against cardio-metabolic risk factors much better than a lacto-ovo-vegetarian diet. So, it appears that the more plant-based a diet is, the more it can help protect against diseases, such as cardiovascular mortality, type-2 diabetes, hypertension, and obesity. Another research done on athletes found that vegan athletes have lower blood pressure compared to athletes who consume animal protein.

Often times when people consider giving up animal products, it seems near impossible. However, it may be easier to let eggs go when you figure out that less than 1 egg per day can increase your risk of heart disease anywhere from 6 to 40%. There is also a 29% increased risk of diabetes! After knowing this, it simply does not seem worth your health to enjoy even half an egg anymore.

Another change that's going to help reduce your risk of cardiovascular disease is going to be including more whole-grain foods! Studies have shown that by including 3 portions of whole-grain foods a day in your diet, you'll be able to reduce the risk of developing cardiovascular disease by lowering your blood pressure. This is nearly as effective as symptom-reducing drugs! Just imagine: you have the power of reducing your risk for these diseases without any of the nasty side effects that come with some of these pharmaceutical drugs.

Along with these small changes, another diet change will be to include flaxseed! Flaxseed is a wonderful little ingredient that has the ability to lower your blood pressure. In one study published in the Journal of Hypertension, researchers found that 1-tablespoon of flaxseed a day has the ability to drop blood pressure by 7 points! In turn, this means that the individual has a 46% lower risk of suffering from a stroke and a 29% lower risk of developing heart disease. Overall, flaxseeds do wonders for our cardiovascular system.

Control and Prevent Cancer

Cancer is a terrible disease that ruins many lives. Luckily, if you change your diet, you have control over preventing cancer. There has been a tremendous amount of research done on this. There is scientific proof that by increasing bean intake by 70g per day, you can cut back on pre-cancer clusters for colon cancer by up to 65%. As you can tell, that is a rather significant number by simply switching your protein intake from an animal product to beans.

Beans contain something known as Inositol hexaphosphate or IP6 for short. Studies have found that

IP6 has the ability to not only prevent cancer in the first place but also control tumor metastasis, progression, and growth. It also appears to have a pretty significant role in overall benefits for our health. IP6 can help to prevent pathological calcification and kidney stone formation. It also enhances the immune system, lowers serum cholesterol levels that have been elevated, and reduces pathological platelet activity. As you can see, beans are almost magical!

If at this point you haven't been persuaded to nix the meat from your diet, I have more science to convince you to take that leap! A study published in the JAMA Internal Medicine Medical Journal has shown that a combined lifestyle of smoking, lack of exercise, and meat consumption can lead to an increased risk of dying from heart disease and cancer. Fat from these animal products can also increase your risk of developing pancreatic cancer by 72%! Pancreatic cancer is the 4th most common cause of death in the world. As you can see, a plant-based diet is so much more than your food choices; it is a simple solution to reclaiming back your health.

Insulin Resistance

As you've learnt earlier, insulin resistance can lead to several different diseases. Science has shown that as you accumulate fat inside of your muscle cells, it would interfere with the action of insulin in your body. Because of the accumulated fat in your muscle cells, the insulin is unable to bring the glucose or sugar from your blood into your muscle, to produce energy.

A high-fat diet can clog your arteries and inhibit insulin from doing its job, thereby increasing insulin resistance levels. The only diet that seems to be able to solve this is a low fat plant-based diet. That's because in general, vegans typically have less fat in their muscles compared to omnivores.

Studies have shown that with a high carb, plant-based diet, some individuals were able to get off their insulin treatment in just 16 days! You might have been told before how terrible carbohydrates are for you and that you should avoid them. However, you'll soon understand that there are healthy carbs you can eat on a plant-based diet and that they can actually combat insulin resistance and make you healthier than ever. The key here is choosing the right carbs, not just any kind of carbs. We will get into that a bit later.

Lower Cholesterol Levels

Many individuals choose to start a plant-based

diet with the intention of lowering their cholesterol levels. A study from The American Journal of Cardiology has shown that coronary artery disease appears nonexistent in cultures where diets are mainly plant-based. This same study has shown that through a plant-based diet, individuals were able to lower and even abolish this disease through diet alone. But, what exactly is in your diet that is causing high cholesterol levels in the first place?

Once again, eggs are the culprit. In a study done on 17 lacto-vegetarian college students, these individuals consumed 400 kcal of foods per day, containing 1 egg for 3 weeks. Another group of individuals followed a similar diet, but without the egg. In the end, the study showed that for those who had 1 egg per day, their cholesterol increased from 97 to 418 mg per day. Just for reference, 200 to 239 mg/dL (milligrams per deciliter) is already considered borderline high for adults.

What then is considered a healthy amount of cholesterol intake? The number is zero. Any intake of trans fats or saturated fats, which by the way can be found in animal products, raises LDL cholesterol concentration. As I've explained earlier, LDL is also known as bad cholesterol. One of the major benefits of a plant-based diet is that you will be able to lower these cholesterol numbers drastically. By doing this, you also increase your overall health.

Reduce Asthma

Asthma is another inflammatory disease that is increasing every year. At this point in time, around 10% of all children suffer from asthma. While it is hard to pinpoint an exact cause, one study has shown that there is a positive correlation between eggs, sweetened beverages, and asthma. Luckily, following a plant-based diet can help lower allergic asthma, due to its higher servings of vegetables and fruits. If children eat 2 servings of vegetables per day, they are 50% less likely to suffer from an asthma attack.

As you can tell, a plant-based diet has a wide number of health benefits, but as I've mentioned earlier, being plant-based is more of a lifestyle compared to just a diet. Yes, the health benefits are wonderful, but it can change your life in other aspects as well! This is exactly why people can stick to a plant-based diet. They see real results. As you gain energy, lose weight, and decrease your risk of disease, you will wonder what took you so long to get started in the first place!

Kick-start Your Plant-Based Lifestyle

Fiber Benefits

When you increase the levels of fruits and vegetables in your diet, you will, in turn, increase the levels of fiber in your diet. In fact, this is one of the top benefits of switching over to a whole food and plant-based diet! Did you know that about 90% of Americans do not reach the daily-recommended amount of fiber? This can lead to health complications and increased risk of colon cancer, breast cancer, heart disease, diabetes, obesity, and stroke. This is because fiber can help control both your blood sugar levels and cholesterol levels. On top of these benefits, fiber also has the ability to bind toxins, mercury, and lead that are found in animal fat, and you can flush them out during excretion. It is like a detox method.

It should be noted that there are two categories of fiber. The first is insoluble fiber. These are the fibers that are made up of plant cells, which are insoluble in water. This is often found in the skins of fruits and seeds. The second is soluble fiber, mostly found in carbohydrates and are in charge of controlling the blood sugar levels in your body. This type of fiber is found in blueberries, beans, nuts and oatmeal.

You will want to increase your fiber benefits

because it can help in a number of key health problems. First, it can help treat moderate diarrhea and prevent constipation. On top of these, fiber also has the ability to help patients who suffer from IBS also known as irritable bowel syndrome. Fiber gives relief to the symptoms that come from irregular stool frequency. It also has the ability to control cholesterol, diabetes, and helps speed up the process of passing food through your intestinal tract!

Antioxidant Benefits

You have probably heard a lot about antioxidants and how beneficial they are for your health. As it turns out, antioxidants seem to work wonders for our body. They have the ability to strengthen the immune system, provide relief from allergies, improve circulation, aid in weight loss, and improve digestion and your quality of sleep. On average, plants contain up to 64 times more antioxidant levels compared to meat. Later, you will learn specific foods that contain antioxidants so that you can include them in your daily diet.

Depression Therapy Benefits

Unfortunately, depression is becoming more prominent in our society today. On average, about 40,000 Americans take their own lives due to depression. Well, on top of reducing the risk of diseases and lowering your body weight, a plant-based diet also helps with mental health issues like anxiety and depression. A study from the Scientific Journal, Nutrition Neuroscience, has shown that consuming foods that are rich in polyphenols could support a healthier mental state. What are polyphenols and where can you get some of them? Polyphenols are natural compounds found commonly in plants and berries. Thus, a plant-based diet has been positively correlated to lower odds of anxiety, depression, and distress due to a higher intake of fruits and vegetables.

Eat Cleaner, Literally

If you still haven't been convinced to cut out meat from your diet by this point, I have more science to persuade you to do so. In the Retail Meat Report by the U.S. Food and Drug Administration FDA, it was reported that 90% of ground beef, ground turkey, and pork chop, and 95% of chicken breasts were contaminated by fecal bacteria. When you imagine yourself putting these products on your cutting board and on your plates, it is just like putting animal feces on them and into your mouth! Even after the animal products were cleaned with detergent and hot water, there were still such high levels of pathogenic fecal bacteria on them.

In a different consumer report, researchers found Yersinia enterocolitica in about 69% of pork samples tested. This is a bacterium that causes illness in about 100,000 Americans per year. 11% of these pork samples were also contaminated with fecal matter. When you think about putting these products into your mouth, it is absolutely revolting.

Weight Loss

Honestly, I could go on for days about the added benefits of the plant-based diet, but it's much more rewarding to experience these benefits for yourself! The final benefit about this diet that I'll include here is weight loss. When you increase your nutritional intake and quality, you'll be able to lose weight like never before. A study published in the Journal of Nutrients has shown that compared to an unrestricted omnivorous diet, a plant-based diet scored higher on its overall nutritional quality.

Weight loss also happens because many plant-based foods are filled with fiber and water, which then helps to keep you satisfied and full for a longer time. So you are less likely to binge and overeat. The second reason why you'll find yourself significantly losing weight all without counting calories is because plant foods tend to be more calorie dense. This means that when you compare 100 calories of broccoli to 100 calories of chicken, people typically have a harder time finishing the portion of broccoli than the chicken. In a nutshell, the plant foods are able to fill you up faster!

As a result, many individuals are able to stick to this diet and enjoy it as a way of life because they no longer need to struggle with cravings or count calories, yet are still able to lose the weight.

Much like any other decision we make in our lives, there'll always be some bad with the good. Obviously, you have just learned that a plant-based diet has some wonderful benefits, but there are some risks that you'll want to be aware of before you begin this diet. Of course, there are ways around these risks, but it is important that you have a full grasp of this diet before starting so that you're able to make informed choices.

Lack of Protein

While I will go over this in greater depth in the next chapter, which addresses all the common misconceptions, a lack of protein is typically a concerned risk of the plant-based diet. As you well know, this diet lacks any type of animal protein, and some see this as a challenge to obtain a proper amount of protein in the diet. When your protein intake is too low, you can't replenish the protein in time while your body is burning up the protein storages in your muscle tissues, and your muscle is where a majority of your calorie burn comes from. As a result, decreased muscle loss could lead to decreased mobility and strength. This typically is only an issue for older folks who truly need the protein to keep them active.

Vitamin B12 Deficiency

A lack of vitamin B12 is another risk that plant-based dieters might have. This is due to the fact that vitamin B12 is mostly present in animal products like dairy, eggs, poultry, and meat. When you follow a plant-based diet, the best solution is to take a supplement to help prevent the deficiency. There are several symptoms of a vitamin B12 deficiency that you'll need to keep an eye out for. These symptoms include memory issues, poor balance, tingling and numbness in extremities, fatigue, and anemia. Of course, these can be easily avoided with regular B12 supplements, but is a risk that should be mentioned, so you are completely aware of all aspects of the plant-based diet.

Iron Deficiency

Another deficiency associated with a plant-based diet is readily absorbable iron. Many individuals who consume a vegetarian diet lack iron-fortified foods. Plant foods have compounds like phytates and oxalates that bind iron to other minerals. When this happens, the iron is unable to be absorbed into the gastrointestinal tract. An example of this would be spinach. Spinach is full of iron, but it cannot be absorbed into our body. On the other hand, poultry or fish can help provide bio-available iron.

The plant-based diet is also known for other mineral deficiencies due to this same issue of decreased absorption. These minerals include selenium, copper, and zinc. Instead, the minerals listed are better absorbed when they come from animal products, which is why plant-based dieters are placed at a slight risk here. Luckily, just like Vitamin B12, a multi-vitamin can help solve this small problem.

Overall, you can easily tell that the good outweighs the bad, especially when the bad can be fixed with a simple supplement. The good news is that a plant-based diet can be altered to fit any person's wants and needs! There are no foods off limits per se, but you can limit or eliminate certain foods depending on what you are trying to accomplish with this diet. Remember, the greatest thing about a plant-based diet is that it is non-restrictive.

In the next chapter, we'll be going over the common misconceptions associated with the plant-based diet. I'm sure you already have many questions pertaining to the plant-based diet, and I am glad you do! Hopefully, within the next few chapters, all of your queries will be answered. As you start this diet, you should expect to be judged and asked a lot of questions. However, stay firm. While there are many misconceptions on the plant-based diet, this next chapter will help clear them up for you!

Chapter Three: Common Misconceptions About the Plant-based Diet

When I first switched over to a plant-based diet, my loved ones seemed to have a hard time supporting my decision. Instead of being excited for me about becoming healthier, I was hit with a million questions about my health. Their reaction was completely understandable as there are indeed many common misconceptions about a plant-based diet. When you first switch over to your new lifestyle, expect to be overwhelmed by the same questions.

In this chapter, we'll be busting the myths associated with a plant-based diet. This way, when your mother asks how you'll be getting your vitamins and proteins, you can reply her with absolute confidence. As you become livelier and start losing weight, people will start to take notice and ask about your lifestyle anyway. So this chapter is created to prepare you to answer all of their questions.

Myth # 1: I have to become Vegan or Vegetarian

As you begin this lifestyle, there is not a single person out there telling you that you need to give up meat! Of course, it all depends on which of the plant-based gurus you follow but becoming plant-based does not mean you need to give up meat entirely. That is why it is called plant-BASED. Some of the plant-based experts out there allow dairy, poultry, fish, and meat in small portions. However, here is my take: at the end of the day, if you are looking to truly benefit from this diet and save the planet, you should eat lesser and smaller portions of meat and then slowly cut them out for good.

One way you can accomplish this is by thinking of meat as a side dish or a treat instead of the main meal. I understand that changing your lifestyle is going to take a lot of work; I have been there! Instead of cutting cold turkey, you can start setting goals for yourself. You could start off by limiting your meat to 2 or 3 times a week. Eventually, you can completely stop eating meat if that is something you wish to do. Again, the last thing that plant-based is, is restrictive. It is a journey, which allows for adjustments. That is what makes it truly different from being strictly a vegan or a vegetarian.

Myth # 2: I have to give up my Snacks

The answer to this is yes and no. Yes, you will be giving up the processed snacks. The snacks that you are used to are probably filled with sugars and oils that are terrible for your health anyway. However, this does not mean that you need to give up snacks for good! Instead, we will begin to focus on creating healthier snacks as replacements. Trust me when I say that you'll never go hungry or have cravings again while on a plant-based diet.

Just because you're on a plant-based diet does not mean that you'll need to deprive yourself. There are plenty of tasty and healthy snacks for you to test out. Some prime examples would be grapes, blueberries, carrot sticks, unsalted nuts, and more! In the final chapter of this book, I'll share with you my top choice for snacks and my personal secret to keeping them on hand.

Myth # 3: Being Plant-based is Too Expensive

This is one of people's favorite arguments! The truth is, eating healthier is going to be much more cost effective when you are smart about your choices. On this diet, you will be eating a lot more whole grains, legumes, and beans. When you compare these with meat and fish prices, they are definitely lower! What's more, these foods are packed with the minerals, vitamins, and protein that your body needs!

There're many economically priced staples you should stock up on such as broccoli, carrots, and leafy greens. If you feel like splurging on your diet, you can go for the "more costly" fruits and vegetables flown in from foreign countries, just for variety of flavors. However, if you want to know how to save money, the secret is to shop for seasonal produce and to do it at the farmers' markets. Not only are the foods there fresher, they tend to be cheaper too!

Lastly, the foods you eat are more filling so you don't even need to purchase the same volume of groceries as before. At the end of the day, would you rather spend more money on healthy foods to keep your body fueled or going to the doctor's for treatment and medicine to fix yourself? I think the answer is pretty clear.

Myth # 4: Eating Plant-based is Boring

We see it in all of the movies; little Johnny

pushing his peas and carrots around because he doesn't want to eat his disgusting vegetables. It isn't until his mother tempts him with a dessert that he will pinch his nose and eat them. Unfortunately, this is the brainwashed mentality that many people carry with them when they think about a plant-based diet. I'm here to tell you that this is simply not the case!

On the plant-based diet, you'll be granted with a huge variety of foods and flavors to help you to be as healthy as possible. In chapter 5, you'll be given an expansive list of foods you can eat on the plant-based diet, and I promise that as long as you are creative, you can make this diet as exciting as possible. It is all about brushing up on your cooking skills so you can make the best out of your diet.

You can say goodbye to your old ways of cooking and hello to exploring new cuisines and styles! Also, you'll most likely discover new vegetables that you never even knew existed. Later in chapter 6, I'll provide you with a meal plan that can work just for you and your whole family. Once you learn how to cook vegetables properly with the right spices, everyone will be asking for seconds. You'll never struggle to eat your vegetables again!

Myth # 5: I Can't Go Out or Eat with Friends

I'm not going to lie; this is one of the more difficult aspects of the plant-based diet. Of course, this depends on whom you surround yourself with. Peer pressure is a real problem among certain groups of friends. Here's an example: you're out with your girlfriends at a restaurant. But when you order a salad, one of them starts shaking her head at you, another one starts to make snide remarks and telling you to get a life. You can expect these kinds reaction A LOT. They are going to happen whether you like it or not; the only thing you have control over is your own reaction. At the end of the day, you know what you want to put into your body, and you understand how beneficial this way of eating is for you. They can do whatever they want with their body; you have to make the best decision for yourself. Just keep this in mind and it's going to help you overcome the peer pressure.

As for the restaurant myth, it simply requires a bit of extra effort from you. In our world today, most restaurants, smaller eateries or fast-food joints typically don't offer plant-based foods. However, that doesn't mean that it is impossible to eat out. Instead, I suggest looking up the menu ahead of time so you know what to expect. There are some wonderful options at restaurants including soups, salads, and pasta that are plant-based. So it is definitely still possible, you'll just have to be more strategic about eating out, and walk in prepared for the situation.

The same rule applies for social events. You should remember that being plant-based doesn't mean that meat is out of the picture for good, but it absolutely should be limited. However, I get it. You still have to live your life! When you're invited to a dinner party or house get-together, there are ways where you can still be respectful and eat what is offered. If you happen to know the host, the best way is to put your request ahead of time for a few vegan or vegetarian dishes. If there are no other options, don't beat yourself up over it. Simply account for it in your food journal and make this one of the nights you eat a little poultry, fish, or meat.

Myth # 6: I am going to feel Deprived and Hungry

One of the major misconceptions about a plant-based diet is that there isn't much to eat on this diet. This is why people think that they'll be hungry all of the time. The truth is, plant-based foods are so high in fiber and protein, that they are the most filling foods out there! As you fill your plate with quinoa, nuts, vegetables, and legumes, you'll be amazed to find that you stay fuller for a longer duration of time.

On top of this, real and whole foods happen to be denser. What this means is they have the ability to keep your body more satisfied on a cellular level, and this is because they are packed with minerals and nutrients. Furthermore, the fruits and vegetables you eat have the ability to decrease blood sugar levels in your body, which then reduces the hunger signals that are sent to your brain. As such, you won't be feeling deprived and hungry all the time.

Myth # 7: I won't get enough Protein

When I first started on my plant-based journey, this was the number one question I was asked. For some reason, there is a myth that you can only get a proper amount of protein if you eat the meat of an animal. However, let me ask you this: how do the pigs, cows and chicken get their protein? From plant sources right? Well, when you're on a plant-based diet, you'll be getting your protein in the same way the animals got it; directly from the plants they eat!

You don't have to worry. There are plenty of different and delicious plant-based ways to meet your daily protein requirements! You have kale, peas, lentils, black beans, quinoa, cashews, almonds, just to name a few. As long as you're eating both a variety and a sufficient amount of plant-based food, you'll get all the essential amino acids to meet the daily protein requirements. What are amino acids? Amino acids are the building blocks of proteins. Understand that your body is a powerful machine; you can actually create your own proteins from amino acids! So this completely debunks the myth that you need animal proteins to get proteins.

Hey! How has this chapter been so far? Has the information been useful enough to help you overcome the many misconceptions about the plant-based diet? I know the protein myth is a big one so I made sure to include it inside this chapter. Let me know if it has helped you by leaving me a short and honest review on Amazon.com. Thank you!

Myth # 8: A Plant-based Diet is Dangerous for Children

If you are like me, you only want the very best for your children. Much like any other diet, food will need to be carefully planned for your kids to make sure they are getting the proper nutrition they need to grow up big and strong. The good news is that a plant-based diet seems to be suitable for any age! Of course, this is taking into account that the right foods are given in the proper quantities.

It is important to note that if you're trying to lose weight on the plant-based diet, your meal choices will probably be high in fiber and low in fat. This particular version of the plant-based diet is not suitable for children. At their age, children are burning a lot of energy and extra calories as they go through their day. If they're being fed too much fiber in their diet, their little stomachs gets filled up fast and they won't have enough space to get more calories. Instead, it is suggested that they go easy on the fiber. Another suggestion is to give them smaller but more frequent meals. Snacking is also an excellent way to ensure a sufficient amount of calories is provided throughout the day.

Myth # 9: Pregnant Women shouldn't eat Plant-Based

Much like with children, women who are expecting a child will need to be very careful with the selection of foods while following a plant-based diet. Luckily, it'll be easy to meet the nutritional needs for two so long as there is proper calorie intake during the second and third trimester. If you're expecting, here are a few particular nutrients you'll need to pay special attention to:

- Calcium

Calcium is a nutrient that is very easy for you to obtain on a plant-based diet because there's a huge selection for it. You have spinach, kale, tofu, soya beans, tahini, almond butter, and fortified non-dairy kinds of milk to choose from. Whether you're pregnant or not, it never hurts to get plenty of calcium.

- Essential Fatty Acids

The key to getting your essential fatty acids is to make sure you're not getting too much omega-6 fatty acids. Instead, focus on consuming soya beans, walnuts, and flaxseed to get the omega-3 fatty acids you need while pregnant.

- Folate and Iron

In the first few weeks of pregnancy, folate is going to be very important. While on a plant-based diet, you can receive folate from foods like oranges, wheat bran, legumes, beans, and leafy greens. Iron-rich foods will also be important along with foods with Vitamin C, which can help to absorb the iron. In order to accomplish this, stick to foods like blackstrap molasses, dried fruits, spinach and sprouts.

- Protein

It is suggested that women who are pregnant up their protein to about 71g per day during the second and third trimester. As we've discussed earlier, you should really have no problem getting your daily protein in as long as you're eating both a variety and sufficient amounts of the right foods. For example, kale, peas, lentils, black beans, quinoa, cashews and almonds.

- Zinc

This is another nutrient that should be increased during pregnancy. Some excellent sources of zinc include cereal, whole grains, legumes, and nuts. To facilitate the absorption of zinc, you can also eat seeds, beans, and sprouted grains. As you can see, just a little knowledge can go a long way to help you get the proper nutrients if you're pregnant.

Myth # 10: I Need to Drink Milk for Strong Bones

We all know the milk commercials; drink milk for strong bones! The truth is, there is not a single person out there who needs to drink cow's milk for strong bones. What you really need is calcium and vitamin D to grow strong bones. Most of the calcium found in our bodies comes from within our bones. When people aren't getting enough calcium, the body then takes the calcium from their bones, which is what weakens them in the first place. If an individual loses too much calcium from his bones, it can, unfortunately, lead to osteoporosis later in life. For this reason, calcium and vitamin D are both super important. Luckily both can be found in abundance while following a plant-based diet.

If you're looking to add calcium into your diet, beans, tofu, plant milk, and dried figs are all excellent sources. As you boost your calcium intake, you'll also want to increase vitamin D to help absorb the calcium into your body. The best way to get vitamin D is to expose yourself to that beautiful weather outside and soak up the sun. However, make sure you do apply sunblock so you don't get the harmful effects of the sunrays. If you live up north and lack constant sunshine in your life, a supplement is always a good alternative.

Myth # 11: I Need to Eat Meat

This statement is so false I cannot even begin to explain it. In fact, the opposite is true, especially after you've read Chapter 2 where I show you the benefits of eating more plants and limiting animal products, and how it affects our planet. Just to repeat, a plant-based diet can help individuals cut their risk of type 2 diabetes, heart disease, certain types of cancer and helps lower cholesterol levels and blood pressure. The research simply does not lie.

You may not know this, but red meat is classified as a Group 1 carcinogen. Do you know what is also in this group? Asbestos and smoking. Most of the meat that you find in the grocery stores has been processed in order to enhance its flavor and improve its preservation. It's also strongly suggested that certain meats cause stomach cancer and colorectal cancer. Research from Cleveland Clinic has found that red meat is linked to clogged arteries. To support this, a study by the American Heart Association also stated that processed meat is linked to heart disease and even increases the risk of heart failure by 8% for every 50 grams.

The real question is why would you risk your health for a piece of animal meat? All of the nutrients you could ever need are already available in a plant-based diet. Not only are the fruits and vegetables delicious, they also prevent certain diseases and can make you feel wonderful inside and out. So to answer the question: no, you do not need to eat meat. Can you? Yes. But should you? Absolutely not.

Myth # 12: Becoming Plant-based is Too Hard

Kick-start Your Plant-Based Lifestyle

The way I look at it, you have a choice. You could carry on with your current diet and just learn to deal with your health issues as they come. Or, you can put in extra effort right now and try a new lifestyle to find out just how incredible you can feel. Much like any new endeavor, it's going to take some work. However, I promise that if you put in the time and effort, you'll enjoy the new experience and even start to recommend it to your friends! Not only will you begin to feel healthier on a plant-based diet, but you will free yourself from cravings and get more energy into your life.

If you're still afraid, I simply ask that you focus on the end goal and just take it one step at a time. As I've mentioned, I've already done all the leg-work on this diet for you and even compiled all of the relevant information you need about a plant-based diet into this book to give you an unfair advantage. I truly want to help you from day one to stick to the diet. After seeing how I've been able to change my life and my children's lives through the plant-based diet, I believe that it's possible for anyone who truly cares about their health. It is going to take work, but it's going to be worth it!

Honestly, I could write a whole other book on the myths and misconceptions of the plant-based diet; but I think you get the point! As you begin this new lifestyle, you should expect questions after questions from those who don't understand it. It is only natural. All you have to remember is this: this is a healthy choice you are making for yourself! It really does not matter what anyone else thinks. It only matters what you believe and what you want for your own health.

With all of this information under your belt, it's now time to learn who the plant-based diet is for. Spoilers Alert: it is great for anybody who wants to be healthy! Whether you have type 2 diabetes, or you are looking to lose weight, or you want to save the planet, there is always a version of the plant-based diet for you.

Chapter Four:
Who is the Plant-based Diet for?

I know I've mostly been addressing people who are trying to get healthy or trying to lose weight for the past 3 chapters. However, even if you're already feeling and looking great and you simply want to take your health to the next level, the plant-based diet is still for you! It should be noted that before you change anything about your diet, you should first discuss your options with a doctor or registered dietitian. Depending on what you're trying to accomplish with your diet, it is possible that there could be a better diet for your specific condition.

On another note, this diet, or any kind of diet is not the best for those who are dealing with or have recently dealt with an eating disorder. This is because there will be major changes made to the quantity and types of foods that you eat. For that reason, it might trigger your history of an eating disorder, and especially if you're still recovering from one. A plant-based diet is meant to make you healthier, but it will take a certain mental capacity to handle the changes. If you've struggled with an eating disorder in the past, please consult a medical professional to create a game plan first before you dive in.

With that being said, this diet can really help those with specific medical conditions. In this chapter, we'll go over some of the reasons how a plant-based diet can help, along with some scientific evidence. At the end of the day, I'm here to show you plants are the way to go, for your health and the environment!

Plant-based Diet for Type 2 Diabetics

In Chapter 2, we touched on how a plant-based diet can help prevent and reverse type 2 diabetes. As the research has shown, meat plays a significant role in the risk for diabetes. Thus, a good way you can protect yourself is by limiting meat and consuming more plant-based foods.

On top of that, in a head-to-head comparison of a plant-based diet versus the diet recommended by the American Diabetes Association, it was proven that it was those on a plant-based diet who showed better results.

They reduced more of their blood sugar, body weight and most importantly, their cardiovascular risk because it's usually the cardiovascular risk that kills a diabetic, whether it is through stroke or heart failure.

In The American Journal of Medicine, there was a study done on a randomized controlled trial group. One of the groups were assigned a plant-based diet with fruits, beans, grains, vegetables, and one portion of low-fat yogurt and limited animal products, while the other group was assigned the official diabetes diet. At the 3 months mark, both groups showed improvements. However, after 6 months, the plant-based diet has pulled ahead and improved their overall quality of life by better controlling their weight, cholesterol, blood sugars, oxidative stress, and insulin sensitivity.

The bottom line is that your diet has an impact on your overall health. It is clear to see that plant-based diet is beneficial, but why? In short, it's got to do with meat. That's why while meat is allowed on a plant-based diet, I strongly encourage you to limit it.

Why is Meat a Risk Factor?

At this point in time, scientists are gaining more and more evidence that there's a link between being obese and having type 2 diabetes. Yet, there hasn't been much attention given to the role of food in this problem. Only recently have they finally started looking into the fact that there's a higher risk for diabetes in those who consume more meat, especially processed poultry.

Unfortunately, there seems to be a rather long list of culprits in meat, so it's hard to narrow down to just one specific reason. Some scientists believe the risk is due to saturated fats, while others think it's animal fat or the trans-fats that are found naturally in animal protein. There are also those who believe it's the heme iron found in meat that is increasing the risk of type 2 diabetes.

However, one thing they can all agree on is that animal-protein is loaded with cholesterol and glycotoxins, which are related to creating inflammation inside your body. Hopefully this long list of potential risks can help you to start limiting the meat in your diet.

How Plants Protect Against Diabetes

As you should know by now, type 2 diabetes is largely due to insulin resistance. Well, free radicals have been discovered to be one of the most important triggers for insulin resistance. In order to combat this, you'll need to consume plant-foods with a lot of antioxidants.

Antioxidants help to boost endogenous antioxidant defenses, and protect against free radicals.

Phytochemicals are found in abundance in many plant foods on the plant-based diet. The good news here is that scientists now believe that these phytochemicals may have the capability to expedite the removal of fat from the organs. This is important because an inflammation of adipose tissues, or fat, is what causes Type 2 Diabetes. Even if it is a low-grade inflammation, it can eventually lead to fatty liver disease and heart disease. I know it seems too good to be true, but eating a plant-based is such a simple way to solve this problem!

On a plant-based diet, fiber is going to become one of your best friends. Studies have shown that fiber can help to decrease insulin resistance by ridding the body of excess estrogen. There's evidence pointing to a direct relationship between diabetes and estrogen. The studies have demonstrated that gut bacteria produce estrogen in our colon. When people followed a high-fat but low-fiber diet, the metabolic activity of the bacteria was stimulated and they over-produce the estrogen in their colon. However, by eating enough fiber, you'll be able to flush out any excess estrogen from your body.

Plant-based Diet for Heart Disease

Unfortunately, heart disease is one of the top causes of deaths. Heart disease begins in childhood, when our arteries slowly begin to harden; this is referred to as atherosclerosis. The plant-based diet might take extra time and effort right now, but in the long run, we're able to slow down or even reverse problems like heart disease and atherosclerosis.

At first, scientists were just hoping to slow down the epidemic of heart disease. However, in a study from The Journal of Family Practice where they placed individuals on a plant-based diet, they were surprised to find that through diet alone, their patients were able to reverse their heart problems. All of this happened as soon as they stopped consuming a diet that was clogging their arteries. In some of the individuals, the plaque actually dissolved away and opened up their arteries, and this is without any surgery or drugs! This proved to the doctors that the body has a way of healing itself when given a chance. The best part of this study was the fact that improvements came through after just a mere 3 weeks!

Making It a Lifestyle

When you think about it, most people don't go to

Kick-start Your Plant-Based Lifestyle

the doctor until there's a problem. The truth is, they could all be prevented through lifestyle alone. By creating a new lifestyle with your plant-based diet, you can help yourself prevent or even reverse the effects of diseases.

In order to live a healthier life, you'll have to remember 4 simple things. First, eat a diet that's based around whole plant foods. Next, stop smoking. There's plenty of research out there about how awful smoking is for you, so I probably don't need to tell you twice. Third, exercise for about half an hour each day. In the final chapter, I'll be sharing some exercise tips to help you get started. Finally, the fourth thing is to get your weight under control. Obese individuals have a higher risk for strokes, cancer, heart attacks and diabetes.

Yes, there are a bunch of medications out there that could help with the issues mentioned earlier, but why complicate things by taking medication? Sometimes, medication could cause allergies and bring on an onslaught of other problems. Instead, changing your lifestyle is a much easier way to do it, and it's completely natural too. As you get used to this lifestyle, your body will start to heal and you'll feel much happier.

Plant-based Diet for Kidney Disease

Kick-start Your Plant-Based Lifestyle

If you're struggling with kidney disease, don't lose hope, because kidney failure can be prevented and treated all through a plant-based diet. Researchers have found that there are currently 3 risk factors for declining kidney function. These risk factors include cholesterol, animal fat and animal protein. As of now, it is believed that animal fat alone can alter the structure of our kidneys by clogging the kidney up.

On top of being able to change the structure of the kidney, animal protein has a major effect on the kidney too. Animal protein has the ability to induce hyperfiltration, meaning that your kidney begins to increase its own workload. The opposite is true for a plant-based diet – our bodies seem to have no adverse reaction with plants. Now the question then is, what is it about animal protein that causes this reaction? The studies have shown that it's because animal protein triggers inflammation.

Along with the inflammation, there is also a terrible acid load that comes with animal foods such as dairy, meat, and eggs. With this much acid in your body, it accumulates in your kidneys, which could eventually lead to tubular toxicity. In simple terms, the acid is damaging the delicate, urine-making tubes that are located within your kidneys. On the other hand, plant-based foods are relatively neutral or even alkaline, and that can even help to counteract the acid.

Treating Chronic Kidney Disease Through Food

If you have kidney disease, you are not alone! In the United States, 1 in 3 adults over the age of 65 have chronic kidney disease. The scary part of this situation is that many individuals do not progress into advanced stages of kidney disease because they typically would have passed away before it started. The real issue connected to kidney disease is heart disease. Indeed, decreasing kidney functions can lead to heart attacks. For this reason, it'll be vital that you choose a diet that helps both your kidneys and your heart. The good news is that the plant-based diet fits both.

As mentioned earlier, a plant-based diet has the ability to protect individuals against heart disease, acidosis, kidney inflammation, kidney stones, and kidney cancer. This can be attributed to the fact that a plant-based diet helps individuals keep their blood pressure under control through vegetables and reduced sodium.

However, there's one potential drawback of the plant-based diet that should be noted. Research has shown that the phosphorus found in meat protein is absorbed more efficiently, at twice the rate compared to plants. The concern here is that when you eat plant-based foods, your phosphorus levels are lower in the blood. For this reason, it will be important that you consult with a professional before beginning a plant-based diet.

Protein and Kidneys

Now, I don't mean to scare you, but 1 in 8 adults have chronic kidney disease without even knowing it. While the progression is slow, the question is what can you do about it? The answer is simple – change your diet! The Western-style diet is the major risk factor associated with chronic kidney disease and impaired kidney function. Through diet, we're impairing the kidney blood flow and creating inflammation that leads to the leakage of protein in the urine.

Two major parts of the average Western-style diet include high-fructose corn syrup and table sugar. Both of these foods are associated with uric acid levels and increased blood pressure, both of which cause major damage to the kidneys. On top of these, there's also cholesterol, trans fat, and saturated fats that are commonly found in a typical Western-style meat-based diet. All these will impact the kidney function as well, which just goes to show that animal protein has a profound negative effect on our kidneys.

Many people believe that an unlimited intake of animal-protein-rich foods is considered normal; this may be one of the most dramatic causes of failing kidney function. While it may have been okay for our predecessors who've had to scavenge for meat in the past, we need to remember that those were during intermittent times. Now, in the modern age and especially in first-world countries, we no longer need to worry about a lack of food sources. Yet, we still have the mentality of the past, consuming an unlimited amount of protein. This would only cause unrelenting stress on our kidneys, eventually leading to scarring and deterioration of the kidneys.

Luckily, plant-protein doesn't have as harsh of an effect on our kidneys. There was a study done on chronic kidney failure patients, where their animal protein was substituted by soya, a plant-protein. The results showed that they experienced less protein leakage and less hyperfiltration. Although this was a short-term study but the important thing to take away from this is that no matter how you look at it, meat seems to affect us more negatively compared to plant-based whole foods.

Kick-start Your Plant-Based Lifestyle

Plant-based Diet for Cancer

Cancer is the second biggest killer of people right behind heart disease. Though the situation looks quite hopeless, studies have shown that not only can a plant-based diet prevent cancer, it can also reverse the effects of certain types of cancer!

There was a study done on the effect of the Standard American Diet on cancer cells; it was found that the average diet could cut down the risk of cancer growth by 9%. However, when these same individuals were placed on a plant-based diet, they cut their risk down by 70% after just 1 year! This specific study was done for prostate cancer, which is the leading killer for men. So what about women? How would a plant-based diet affect breast cancer? Well, after 2 weeks of being on a plant-based diet, 3 different types of breast cancer were found to have reduced drastically. By the end, scientists found that only a few cancer cells remained in the blood test. They also found that the bloodstream became much more effective in protecting you against cancer, all due to a simple diet change.

While slowing down the growth of these cancer cells is a nice concept; getting rid of them altogether is even better. This process is known as apoptosis or programmed cell death. When an individual eats healthy, the body gains the ability to reprogram cancer cells and forces them into retirement. With a plant-based diet, you can teach your body to slow down and stop cancer cell growth in as little as 2 weeks!

Fruits and Cancer

If you know that diet can help slow and get rid of cancer, it's important to understand what foods you can eat. Fruits are going to be vital on a plant-based diet whether for health reasons or not. A study published in the Journal of Agricultural and Food Chemistry was done on the effectiveness of 11 common fruits on cancer cells.

When the cancer cells start out at 100% growth, pineapples, pears, and oranges seemed to have a minor effect. Peaches appeared to have a higher effect, but the greatest defenders to cancer cells were bananas and grapefruits. These two fruits were able to drop the growth rate of cancer by 40%! Along with these two fruits, apples, strawberries, and red grapes are also really effective. These 3 fruits are able to cut cancer cells by half!

As I've mentioned at the start of this chapter, a plant-based diet can benefit a variety of people. I now want to take the time to list a few more people who can benefit from this diet, although do note that it's not the complete list. Ok here we go, the plant-based diet is beneficial for any individual who has:

- Lung Disease
- Brain Disease
- Digestive Cancer
- Infections
- High Blood Pressure
- Parkinson's Disease
- Suicidal Depression
- Blood Cancer
- Liver Disease

If you're looking to fight any of these diseases or simply want to better your health, the plant-based diet will be perfect for you.

As you know, it's going to take a certain amount of work. Unfortunately, if this were easy, everyone would already be doing it. However, you are different. You have an unfair advantage. You know the science behind it that proves that it works. Now, you just have to put in the work. As you go through the motions, it will become easier and easier!

The next chapter coming up is where you'll learn all the delicious foods you can enjoy on the plant-based diet,

Kick-start Your Plant-Based Lifestyle

along with the ones that you should limit or avoid.

Chapter Five: Foods to Enjoy and Avoid on a Plant-based Diet

Now, we get to the fun part! If you still believe that a plant-based diet is going to be restrictive, be prepared to have your mind changed forever. The truth is, the plant-based diet includes a wide variety of foods that you get to enjoy. I know so many people who enjoy this diet and the benefits that go along with it; isn't it about time you join them?

To start off, we'll go over all of the incredible foods that you'll be enjoying. After that, we'll go in depth on the foods you should avoid on the plant-based diet. As mentioned earlier, there's a misconception that plant-based means no meat. That's wrong. You can still have the meat. However, after reading about the troubles it can cause to your health and our dear planet, you might want to limit it or even give it a miss. Once you have everything you need to know, be sure to read the next chapter where I've created an expandable grocery list for you, some delicious recipes and even a simple meal plan to help you get started. I want to give you as much help as possible so success is closer than you think in your plant-based journey.

Foods to Eat Freely

One of the major benefits of the plant-based diet is that you can say goodbye to calorie counting! I mentioned earlier that the foods you'll be eating will be much more calorie-dense, meaning that you'll feel fuller more easily and for a longer time! You can say goodbye to counting calories and hello to actually enjoying your food! To begin, we will go over the foods that you can consume freely.

Fruits

While all fruits are allowed, it should be noted that not all fruits are created equal. Each fruit provides its own unique health benefits and coming right up, you will get my compilation of some of the healthiest fruits for your plant-based diet.

- <u>Cranberries</u>

Cranberries are unique fruits that are rich in vitamin K1, vitamin E, manganese, vitamin C, and copper! They also have a significant number of antioxidants that improve health significantly. Cranberries also contain A-type proanthocyanidins, which research has shown, to be a great help in preventing gum inflammation and urinary tract infections.

- <u>Strawberries</u>

Strawberries are among the most recommended fruits. On top of being delicious, it is also full of potassium, folate, manganese, and vitamin C. When compared to other fruits, strawberries are considered to have a low glycemic index, meaning they won't cause blood sugar spikes. A study published in the Anticancer Research journal has found that strawberries can actually prevent tumor growth.

- <u>Mango</u>

Mango is an excellent fruit to add to your fruit list, especially in the summertime! Mango has soluble fiber and provides vitamin C, which makes it anti-inflammatory. It also has strong antioxidants that lower the risk of diseases. In animal studies, it was found that the compounds in mangos could help protect against diabetes.

- <u>Pomegranate</u>

If you haven't had pomegranates before, you're missing out! Pomegranates are nutrient dense and have an excellent level of antioxidants to keep you healthy. In fact, a study published in the Journal of Agricultural and Food Chemistry has found that pomegranate juice has 3 times higher levels of antioxidants compared to red wine and green tea! On top of this, it's also full of different kinds of polyphenols, which reduces the chance of developing cancer.

- <u>Apples</u>

We have all heard it, an apple a day keeps the doctor away. As it turns out, there seems to be some truth to the saying! Apples are very nutritious and contain high amounts of vitamin K, potassium, vitamin C, and fiber! They also provide B vitamins. Research has shown that antioxidants found in apples can help promote heart health and may reduce the risk of Alzheimer's, cancer, and type 2 diabetes.

- <u>Blueberries</u>

Blueberries are most commonly known for their high levels of antioxidants, but they are also high in manganese, vitamin K, vitamin C and fiber! Jam-packed with all these nutrients, it's no wonder blueberries can help reduce the risk of certain chronic conditions including diabetes and heart disease.

- <u>Pineapple</u>

With just one cup of this delicious fruit, you receive all of the vitamin C you need for the day, plus a hefty amount of manganese too. Pineapple also has bromelain, which helps to digest proteins. In addition, studies have proven that pineapples can help fight and protect against cancer and tumor growth.

- <u>Grapefruit</u>

The list of fruits you can enjoy goes on and on, but I'll end off with grapefruit. Grapefruit is one of the healthiest citrus fruits out there and is an excellent source of the vitamins and minerals. Research shows that grapefruit is associated with reduced cholesterol levels and may help prevent the forming of kidney stones.

Vegetables

On a plant-based diet, the bulk of what you'll be eating will be vegetables. Obviously, this does not come as a surprise. There are plenty of vegetables for you to enjoy, but the following are the real powerhouses that you'll want to include as often as possible into your diet.

- <u>Brussels Sprouts</u>

Brussels sprouts are one of those vegetables that you absolutely love or loathe. The truth is, it is all in the preparation! Brussels sprouts contain an antioxidant known as kaempferol. This specific antioxidant is linked to the prevention of any cell damage that is caused by oxidative stress, and is an important antioxidant to keep chronic diseases at bay. Additionally, brussels sprouts are an excellent source of potassium, manganese, folate, and vitamin C, A and K!

- <u>Garlic</u>

Rejoice all my garlic lovers! Garlic has many roots in our history as a medicinal plant. One of its main active compounds is allicin, and the research has shown that this compound helps to regulate blood sugar and promotes excellent heart health. It was also found in a study published in *The American Journal of Clinical Nutrition* that garlic is beneficial in lowering total blood cholesterol, LDL cholesterol, and triglycerides, all while increasing healthy HDL cholesterol.

- <u>Broccoli</u>

Broccoli is a part of the cruciferous family. This vegetable is rich in vitamin C and vitamin K. It also contains an abundant amount of potassium, manganese, and folate, which we need daily. Broccoli also contains sulforaphane, which has been found to have a protective effect against cancer. In one specific study, sulforaphane was successfully able to reduce the number and size of breast cancer cells while simultaneously blocking tumor growth.

- <u>Carrots</u>

In one cup of carrots, you'll receive 428% of your daily recommended vitamin A. Carrots also contain the antioxidant beta-carotene which is associated with cancer prevention. In fact, one study found that by eating one serving of carrots during a week could lower the risk of prostate cancer by 5%.

- <u>Spinach</u>

Of course, spinach is on the list! Spinach tops the charts as being one of the healthiest vegetables, and it isn't hard to understand why! Spinach is rich in iron, vitamin A, vitamin K, and is also packed with antioxidants. It also contains the compound called carotenoid, which the research has shown, can help individuals reduce their risk of cancer.

Legumes

While beans and legumes are more known for their fiber and B vitamins, they're also the main source of protein for your new, plant-based diet. Now, I will list some of the healthier ones you should make into staples, or when you're looking to switch out those animal proteins.

- <u>Black Beans</u>

Black beans might just become one of your new favorite foods. Not only are they packed with fiber and folate, they also offer 15.2 grams of protein in just one cup! These beans are beneficial as they have a lower glycemic index when compared to other foods with higher carbohydrates content. This means they can help control your blood sugar levels while being eaten as a staple. Scientists have even found evidence that black beans can help individuals manage their weight and type 2 diabetes.

- <u>Kidney Beans</u>

These beans are another food that is fairly common on a plant-based diet. Comparable to black beans, a cup of kidney beans contains an impressive 13.4 grams of protein. They are also high in fiber and are known to help slow down the absorption of sugar into the bloodstream. In the same study mentioned earlier, it was found that there is a connection between kidney beans and type 2 diabetes as well. On top of that, the fiber in kidney beans also helped to reduce the spike in blood sugar after finishing a meal.

- <u>Peas</u>

Peas are an excellent source of protein and fiber. They also have the ability to reduce insulin and blood sugar after a meal. What's more, you're not restricted to just plain peas anymore. Now, there is something called pea starch and it's also good for you. In fact, there is a study from the European Journal of Nutrition that discovered that pea starch could help you feel fuller for a longer amount of time.

- Lentils

The next time someone asks how you get your protein on a plant-based diet, you'll know the answer is lentils. In one cup of lentils, you'll get a whopping 17.9 grams of protein! The research has shown that eating lentils helps to reduce blood sugar and lower the risk of diabetes. Another study published in The American Journal of Clinical Nutrition has even shown that lentils can improve gut health by increasing your bowel function. When the stomach is emptied at a quicker rate, digestion increases and spikes in blood sugar is prevented.

- Chickpeas

The final source of protein that makes my list is chickpeas. They are often referred to as garbanzo beans and make an excellent source of fiber and protein. In one cup of chickpeas, you'll get 14.5 grams of protein. Specifically, chickpeas are great for reducing blood sugar levels and increasing sensitivity to insulin. It should also be noted that chickpeas can help improve bowel movement, by reducing the level of bad bacteria stuck in your intestines.

Whole Grains

As you switch to a plant-based diet, grains are going to become another staple in your household. Firstly, there are 3 types of whole grains – the bran, the germ, and the endosperm. Each one of these has its own nutrients, which are vital for your health. Whole grains are excellent as they are high in dietary fiber, B vitamins, selenium, phosphorus, manganese, magnesium, and iron! Here, I will share with you some of my favorites!

- <u>Quinoa</u>

In South America, quinoa is a superfood! This is because this grain is packed with fiber, healthy fats, proteins and all the minerals and vitamins you need for a well-rounded diet. A study has shown that quinoa also contains the antioxidant kaempferol, (just like Brussels sprouts) and it helps in the prevention of certain types of cancers, heart disease and chronic inflammation.

- <u>Brown Rice</u>

For a majority of you, up until this point in your life, you've mostly been eating white rice. Yet, brown rice is the healthier alternative. This is because brown rice is a whole grain – it still has the bran and germ intact, which makes it richer in fiber, antioxidants, minerals, and vitamins. Along with these benefits, brown rice also happens to be gluten-free, which makes it an excellent choice if you need to follow a gluten-free diet.

- Whole-grain Bread

On top of switching from white rice to brown rice, you'll also want to consider switching from white bread to whole-grain bread. There's a wide variety including whole-grain tortillas, bagels, rolls, and rye bread. Although it's a simple switch, you're actually adding more whole grains into your diet and this is extremely nutritious.

Foods to Limit

In this next section, I will list off the foods you should still eat, but in sparing amounts. This means that even though they're allowed and do provide great health benefits, it doesn't mean you should eat them every day. That's because they also add a high amount of fat into your diet. This is especially crucial if you're looking to lose weight.

- Avocado

I said the same thing you're probably saying to yourself

right now: Avocado is a fruit? Indeed, it is, but they are very different from your typical fruit. While most fruits are high in carbohydrate, avocado is low in carbs and acts more as an excellent source of healthy fats. The nutrients found in avocado include monounsaturated fat and oleic acid, both of which research has shown to be associated with better heart health and reduced inflammation.

- <u>Nuts & Nut Butters</u>

Nuts are also an excellent source of fiber and protein. They are also commonly used as a healthy snack option. However, they do contain a relatively high fat content. The fat found in nuts include monounsaturated fat, omega-6, and omega-3 polyunsaturated fat. It should be noted that these fats are considered healthy, but you'll still want to consume them in moderation.

Examples: Peanut Butter, Tahini. Cashew Butter, Almond Butter, Walnuts, Pistachios, Pecans, Peanuts, Coconut, Cashews, Almonds.

- <u>Seeds & Seed Butters</u>

Just like nuts; seeds are a great snacking alternative. Seeds are extremely nutritious and are an excellent source of fiber. They could potentially help to lower your blood pressure, cholesterol levels, and blood sugar. However, it's true that there can be too much of a good thing. So, although seeds contain polyunsaturated fats and healthy monounsaturated fats, which are essentially good fats, they should still be limited. Examples: Sunflower Seeds, Sesame Seeds, Flaxseeds, Chia Seeds.

- <u>Beverages</u>

It should be noted that water is going to be the best beverage for you, but it is completely understandable if you don't want to just drink water for the rest of your life. This is why the following beverages are allowed, but should be limited to only a few times per week.

1. Fruit Juices
2. Unsweetened Plant Milk, eg. Soy Milk or Almond Milk
3. Processed Smoothies
4. Soy Yogurt

- <u>Dried Fruits</u>

Dried fruits are more processed compared to their whole or raw versions. If you do include dried fruits in your diet, you'll want to make sure that they are unsulfured. Some examples of dried fruits you could try include: Raisins, Medjool Dates, Currants, Cherries, Blueberries, Apricots, or Apples.

- <u>Sweeteners</u>

Adding a little sweetener is the secret ingredient to making yummy desserts or to satisfy your sweet tooth. However, you'll want to choose those that are minimally processed. I suggest looking for maple sugar, date sugar, or even cane sugar. On top of these options, you can always choose pure maple syrup. The goal is to make sure that you're getting real maple syrup and not something that is maple-flavored. These are very important differences you'll want to be conscious of when you start a plant-based diet.

- <u>Condiments</u>

When it comes to condiments, you'll need to be selective as well. While there are plenty of options on the market, you'll still want to select condiments that are going to be compliant with your new diet. Some of my favorites include Hot Sauce, Wasabi Paste, Vegan Worcestershire Sauce, Apple Cider Vinegar and Tomato Sauce. In the next chapter, you'll be gifted with a thorough grocery list to help you get started on your new diet!

Foods to Avoid

Here is where it might get tough for some of you. At the end of the day, it is important to remember this phrase: "do not let the food control you." You are in control. You are the only person who can decide what goes into your body. The question is this, "do you want to fuel your body with nutrients or clog it up with unhealthy foods?" While it may take some work at first, you'll soon get used to it and naturally avoid these foods!

- <u>Animal-based Foods</u>

This is a given but remember that it isn't absolutely restricted! You SHOULD avoid them, but if you feel you absolutely need an animal protein, it is allowed in small portions. Some of the animal-based proteins you should avoid include fish, shellfish, game meats, chicken, turkey, pork, lamb, and beef. We have already gone over why meat might not be the best for your health, so how much of it you would allow in your diet is a decision you'll have to make for yourself.

- <u>Eggs</u>

This is another food that is tough for some people at the beginning. You'd be surprised to know that eggs are included in so many different types of foods. Whether it's your favorite bread or muffin, you'll want to avoid eggs (egg whites included). While it may be difficult in the beginning, it is absolutely possible to avoid them. So don't give in.

- Dairy

You'll want to avoid dairy while on the plant-based diet. This includes foods such as cream, yogurt, butter, cheese, and milk. You'll also need to be mindful of any food that contains a dairy product, or an ingredient made from a dairy product. As long as it is coming from an animal, like sheep, goats or cows, it should be avoided. Luckily, there're plenty of plant-based alternatives to keep you satisfied. Some examples are soymilk, cashew cheese, tofu yogurt, coconut whipped cream and frozen banana ice cream!

- Artificial & Refined Foods

Remember that this diet is all about consuming foods that are plant-based. From this point on, you will want to avoid foods that contain chemical additives such as preservatives, flavorings, or colorings. You'll also want to avoid any foods that have refined sugars or bleached flour. In the tips and tricks chapter, you'll be learning everything you need to know about reading a food label to help you avoid these ingredients. It can be tricky at first, but with some effort, you can say goodbye to artificial foods forever.

- <u>Oils</u>

If you are looking to lose weight, this is going to be a big factor for you! When you follow a plant-based diet, you'll be saying goodbye to any type of extracted oils. This includes fish oil, coconut oil, vegetable oil, and even olive oil! If you're like me, you would probably be wondering what you're going to cook with if you can't use oil. Don't worry, you'll soon find out once you get into the recipes section in the next chapter!

I understand this might be a lot to take in at once right now and I don't blame you if you feel a bit overwhelmed. However, I'm determined to provide you this information so as to give you a head start. By now, you should've understood the gist of it – whole foods are good; artificial foods are bad. The essential nutrients we need are found in both animals and plants, so why not choose the one that comes from plants? All you have to do is get used to its taste.

In the next chapter, you'll be provided with a grocery list, recipes and a simple meal plan to help you get started. As you learn more about the foods you enjoy, you'll be able to expand upon what I've given you. I hope that by the end of this book, you'll be confident enough to

Kick-start Your Plant-Based Lifestyle

start your journey and better your health. Now let's move onto the next chapter and get cooking!

Chapter Six: Grocery List and Meal Plan

Finally, we get to the fun part: eating! Because I want to set you up for complete success on your plant-based diet, I've created a meal plan along with the exact recipes you'll need to follow through. Don't worry they are beginner level and easy to fix up, so I hope you're ready to prepare some delicious plant-based foods.

At the end of the chapter, you'll also have the complete grocery list, which includes the ingredients needed for all the recipes and other foods you'll be able to enjoy while on the plant-based diet.

Breakfast Recipes

1. Oat Waffles

Time: 30 Minutes

Servings: 12 Waffles

Ingredients:

- Mashed Bananas (.33 C.)
- Unsweetened Almond Milk (1.50 C.)
- Ground Cinnamon (.50 t.)
- Grated Lemon Zest (2 t.)
- Ground Flaxseeds (.25 C.)
- Rolled Oats (2.50 C.)
- Sliced Bananas (Optional)

Directions:

1. It should first be noted that you'd need a waffle iron for this recipe. When you acquire one, warm it up so it will be hot and ready!

2. Next, take out a medium bowl and mix together the cinnamon, lemon zest, flaxseeds, and oats. Once this is complete, place the ingredients into a blender and blend at a high power until a powdery consistency is created.

3. With the powder created, place it back into your bowl. Now, you'll want to stir in the mashed banana

and almond milk. When you are finished mixing everything together, the batter should be fairly thick.

4. Finally, you're going to pour the batter into your waffle iron machine and cook according to its directions. Repeat with the remaining batter.

5. Lastly, once all of them are done cooking, serve with some sliced bananas for extra flavor.

Kick-start Your Plant-Based Lifestyle

2. Plant-based Breakfast Burrito

Time: 60 Minutes

Servings: 4 Burritos

Ingredients:

- Whole-grain Tortillas (4)
- Nutritional Yeast (.25 C.)
- Extra-firm Tofu (1 Lb.)
- Dried Thyme (1 t.)
- Garlic Cloves (3)
- Ground Turmeric (2 t.)
- Dried Basil (2 T.)
- Chopped Red Bell Pepper (1 C.)
- Chopped Onion (1 C.)
- Chopped Sweet Potato (1 C.)
- Salt & Pepper (To Taste)

Directions:

1. To start this recipe, you'd first want to heat your oven to 350 degrees. As this warms up, you can begin to heat up a large skillet and cook your bell peppers, onions, and sweet potatoes for about 10 minutes. If your vegetables begin to stick to your pan, try to add water 1 tablespoon at a time to help.

2. Once the vegetables are cooked through, you can add the turmeric, basil, dried thyme and your garlic

cloves into the skillet. You will want to cook all these ingredients for about a minute and then stir in the nutritional yeast and extra-firm tofu. If desired, you can use this time to season with salt and pepper as well.

3. When these two steps are completed, transfer everything into a baking pan and bake for 35 minutes, or until the tofu turns a nice light brown. It will be helpful to turn everything over occasionally, so it cooks through.

4. Finally, you'd want to carefully spoon your tofu mixture into your tortillas. Once all of the ingredients are in place, fold your tortilla, roll and enjoy breakfast.

3. Stuffed Sweet Potato

Time: 30 Minutes

Servings: 1

Ingredients:

- Hemp Seeds (1 T.)
- Fresh Berries (.25 C.)
- Rolled Oats (3 T.)
- Almond Butter (1 T.)
- Baked Sweet Potato (1)
- Maple Syrup (1 t.)

Directions:

1. First, heat up your oven to 425 degrees. Then cook the sweet potatoes for 15 to 18 minutes. Halfway through the cooking time, you should flip them over so that all the potatoes cook through.

2. Once the potato is cooked through, carefully remove it from the oven and slice it in half. When the potato is cool enough to handle, take a spoon and scoop the flesh out of each half.

3. Next, place the sweet potato flesh into a bowl and combine with the maple syrup and almond butter. You can also add a pinch of salt for flavor and then stir to combine everything together well.

4. After that, return the mixture into the shell of the

Kick-start Your Plant-Based Lifestyle

sweet potato. Now, I invite you to use your creativity with the toppings for this. For my stuffed potatoes, I love to add cooked oats, hemp seeds, and berries. The options are truly endless; just be sure you stick with plant-based ingredients.

5. For extra flavoring, serve with maple syrup, but make sure it is pure and not maple-flavored.

4. Overnight Oats

Time: 8 Hours

Servings: 1

Ingredients:
- Cinnamon (.25 t.)
- Unsweetened Maple Syrup (1 T.)
- Water (.50 C.)
- Unsweetened Plant Milk (Soy or Almond) (.25 C.)
- Rolled Oats (.75 C.)
- Vanilla Extract (.10 t.)
- Fresh Berries (Optional)
- Chia Seeds (1 T.) (Optional)

Directions:

1. Not only is this breakfast extremely easy, but it is also very delicious! To start, get yourself a jar that has an airtight lid. Once this is obtained, go ahead and pour in the oats, followed by the water and plant milk.

2. Next, add in the vanilla, cinnamon and maple syrup. When everything is in place, stir the ingredients to make sure it is well blended. Once that is done, seal the jar and place in the fridge overnight.

3. For your breakfast the next morning, remove from the fridge and enjoy your overnight oats. For some extra flavor, feel free to add in any plant-based foods

that you like! For my personal overnight oats, I add chia seeds and fresh berries for some extra sweetness.

5. Black Bean and Corn Cake

Time: 35 Minutes

Servings: 10 Cakes

Ingredients:

- Sliced Green Onions (6)
- Cooked Black Beans (1 C.)
- Frozen Corn Kernels (1 Package)
- Diced Red Bell Pepper (1)
- Unsweetened Applesauce (.25 C.)
- Unsweetened Plant Milk (1.50 C.)
- Salt (.50 t.)
- Baking Powder (1 T.)
- Cornmeal (.50 C.)
- Whole Wheat Pastry Flour (1.50 C.)

Directions:

1. Before you begin cooking, you'd first want to heat your oven to 200 degrees.

2. As the oven warms up, take a bowl and combine the salt, baking powder, cornmeal, and flour together. Once this step is complete, carefully create a well in the flour.

3. In the well, carefully pour in the applesauce and your plant milk of choice. Once these are in place, add in the green onions, black beans, corn, and bell

pepper. Then fold all of the ingredients together but be sure not to overmix as it might activate the baking powder.

4. Next, you'll need to heat up a nonstick pan over a medium heat. When it is warm enough, spoon a half cup of batter onto the pan to create your pancake. Go ahead and cook each cake until they are crisp around the edges and then flip. Each side of the pancake should take around 5 minutes.

5. Once the pancakes are cooked, transfer them to a platter and pop in the oven for around 10 minutes. By the end, the cakes should be nice and crispy!

Lunch Recipes

1. Red Pepper and Tomato Soup

Time: 45 Minutes

Servings: 8 Cups

Ingredients:

- Unsweetened Plant Milk (1 C.)
- Black Pepper (.10 t.)
- Salt (50 t.)
- Chopped Oregano (1 t.)
- White Wine Vinegar (1 T.)
- Diced Carrots (1 C.)
- Diced Green Beans (1 C.)
- Whole Grain Penne (2 C.)
- Garlic Cloves (3)
- Wedged Onion (1)
- Chopped Red Bell Pepper (3 C.)
- Chopped Tomatoes (5 C.)

Directions:

1. To start this delicious soup, you'll first want to heat your oven to 425 degrees. As it warms up, you can go ahead and prepare a baking sheet by lining it with parchment paper.

2. Once this is completed, carefully place the garlic,

onion, bell pepper, and tomatoes onto your baking sheet. When everything is in place, cook the vegetables in the oven for 30 minutes.

3. As the vegetables bake, fill up a pot with water to prepare cooking your penne. Place the pot on the stovetop and bring the water to a boil. Once boiling, add in your carrots, green beans, and whole grain penne. You will want to cook the penne according to the package's instructions and add in the peas 2 minutes before it is done. When these have been cooked through, drain away the water and put everything else to the side.

4. Next, remove the vegetables from the oven. Once they're cool enough to handle, put your roasted vegetables into a blender along with a cup of water, pepper, salt, oregano, and the white wine vinegar. Then, blend on high until the ingredients create a nice, smooth soup.

5. Now pour the soup into a pot and bring everything to a boil. Once it is boiling, add in your carrots, green beans, penne, and plant milk. Go ahead and cook everything for 4 to 5 minutes and then your soup will be ready for lunch!

2. White Bean and Cauliflower Creamy Soup

Time: 1 Hour

Servings: 8 Cups

Ingredients:

- Cannellini Beans (1 Can)
- Cauliflower Florets (4 C.)
- Garlic Cloves (4)
- White Miso Paste (4 t.)
- Chopped Onion (1 C.)
- Cubed and Peeled Potatoes (4 C.)
- Black Pepper (.10 t.)
- Chopped Scallions & 1 lemon wedge (Optional)

Directions:

1. To make this delicious, nutrient-packed soup, pour 4 cups of water along with the garlic, miso, onion, and potatoes into a pot. When all of these ingredients are in place, bring everything to a boil and then reduce to a medium-low heat.

2. When the ingredients are simmering, cover the pot with a tightly fitted lid and cook everything for 25 minutes.

3. Once the vegetables are cooked through, you can turn off the heat and allow the ingredients to cool

slightly. When it is safe to handle, transfer the soup over to a blender and blend on high until everything is nice and smooth with a creamy consistency.

4. Next, you'd want to transfer the soup back into your pot. Once in place, you can go ahead and add in the cauliflower and beans.

5. Now, bring everything to a boil over a high heat. Once it is boiling, reduce to a medium heat. Then, place the cover on and simmer everything for 12 minutes. By then, the cauliflower should be tender.

6. Finally, portion out your soup and enjoy! For extra flavor, try adding pepper, scallions, and even a nice, fresh lemon wedge!

Kick-start Your Plant-Based Lifestyle

3. Stuffed Lettuce Cups

Time: 15 Minutes

Servings: 15

Ingredients:

- Romaine Lettuce Hearts (15)
- Fresh Lime Juice (3 T.)
- Grated Lime Zest (1 t.)
- Chili Powder (1 T.)
- Chopped Jalapeno Pepper (1)
- Chopped Red Bell Pepper (.50 C.)
- Halved Cherry Tomatoes (1 C.)
- Chopped Mango (1)
- Black Beans (1 Can)
- Corn Kernels (2 C.)
- Sliced Avocado (1) (Optional)
- Hot Sauce (Optional)

Directions:

1. For a quick, simple lunch, simply take all of the ingredients from the list and mix them well in a bowl. If desired, you can go ahead and season with salt and pepper according to your taste.

2. Then peel the Romaine Hearts into individual leaves.

3. Once everything is well mixed, spoon it into your lettuce leaf and lunch is served! For extra flavor, add some slices of avocado and drizzle some hot sauce!

4. Spicy Potato Bowl

Time: 35 Minutes

Servings: 4

Ingredients:

- Fresh Spinach (4 C.)
- Chopped Scallions (2)
- Diced Red Bell Pepper (1)
- Frozen Corn (8 Oz.)
- Diced Tomatoes and Green Chilies (1 C.)
- Pinto Beans (1 Can)
- Potatoes (4)
- Cilantro (Optional)
- Hot Sauce (Optional)

Directions:

1. Before you put together your salad, you will first need to cook your potatoes. You can do this whichever way you prefer – whether you pop them into the microwave for 10 minutes or in the oven at 375 degrees for one hour. By the end, the potato needs to be cooked through.

2. Next, cook the pinto beans. Once cooked through, take a fork and smash them. Once this step is completed, go ahead and add in the green onion,

pepper, corn, tomatoes and green chilies. Be sure to mix everything together well so the flavor will be spread across evenly.

3. Now, take your salad bowls and place a layer of fresh spinach at the bottom. Then put a layer of potato, and finally, topped it off with the bean mixture. For extra flavor, you can add in cilantro and some hot sauce.

5. White Bean Hash

Time: 30 Minutes

Servings: 4

Ingredients:

- Kale (1 C.)
- White Cannellini Beans (2 C.)
- Diced Sweet Potato (1)
- Minced Rosemary (2 t.)
- Minced Garlic (3)
- Diced Red Bell Pepper (1)
- Chopped Leek (1)
- Juice and Zest of Orange (1)
- Salt & Pepper (To Taste)

Directions:

1. To start off, you will want to take a large saucepan and heat it over a medium heat. Once it is warm, you can add in the red pepper and leek. Go ahead and cook these two ingredients for 8 to 10 minutes. If the vegetables are sticking to the pan, try adding 1 tablespoon of water at a time to prevent this from happening.

2. Once the vegetables are cooked through, add in the rosemary and garlic and cook everything together

for another minute or so. After that, you can add in the orange zest, orange juice, beans, and sweet potato. When these ingredients are in place, cook for 10 minutes or until the vegetables become nice and tender.

3. Finally, you're going to add in the kale and cook for another 5 minutes. For extra flavor, add salt and pepper to taste. When you are ready for your meal, divide into portions and enjoy!

Dinner Recipes

1. Lemon Dijon Cauliflower

Time: 1.5 Hour

Serving: 1 Cauliflower

Ingredients:

- Red Pepper Flakes (.25 t.)
- Ground Turmeric (.25 t.)
- Fresh Parsley (.25 C.)
- Nutritional Yeast (2 T.)
- Minced Garlic (3)
- Lemon Juice (3 T.)
- Dijon Mustard (2 T.)
- Cauliflower (1)

Directions:

1. To start, heat your oven to 425 degrees. As it warms up, you will want to prepare your cauliflower by cutting the stem off.

2. Next, take out your blender and place the following inside: red pepper flakes, turmeric, parsley, nutritional yeast, garlic, lemon juice, and Dijon mustard. Once in place, blend everything until the ingredients are smooth.

3. With the sauce created, carefully brush the

cauliflower with one-third of the sauce. When this is completed, place the bowl of sauce to the side for later use.

4. Put your cauliflower into a Dutch oven, place the lid on, and roast your cauliflower in the oven for 30 minutes.

5. Remove the Dutch oven from the oven and brush the sauce over the cauliflower again. Then Repeat Step 4.

6. After another 30 minutes has passed, cover the cauliflower with the remaining of the sauce and roast it for another 10 minutes, but this time, without the Dutch oven lid on.

7. Finally, remove the Dutch oven from the oven and dinner is served. For extra flavor, try topping the cauliflower with extra red pepper flakes.

Kick-start Your Plant-Based Lifestyle

2. Penne and Cheese

Time: 45 Minutes

Servings: 2

Ingredients:

- Whole Grain Penne (4 Oz.)
- Salt (1 t.)
- Nutritional Yeast (.50 C.)
- Water (2 C.)
- Raw Cashews (.50 C.)
- Minced Garlic (2)
- Ground Turmeric (1 t.)
- Chopped Onion (.50 C.)
- Chopped Carrots (1 C.)
- Cubed Potato (1)

Directions:

1. To start, you will want to mix water, garlic, turmeric, onions, carrots, and potatoes into a saucepan. When everything is in place, go ahead and bring everything to a boil and then reduce to a lower heat. When this is done, reduce the heat to a simmer for 20 minutes.

2. As these ingredients cook, you will want to begin soaking the cashews. Allow these to soak for at least

10 minutes.

3. While the cashews are soaking, cook your pasta according to the directions on its packaging. After the cashews have soaked for at least 10 minutes, drain the water.

4. Next, add the cashews, half a cup of water, nutritional yeast and the potato mixture into your blender. Go ahead and blend all of these ingredients together for 2 minutes or so. By the end, you should have a nice and creamy sauce.

5. Finally, pour the sauce over the pasta, and you have just made yourself a delicious mac and cheese for dinner!

3. Sloppy Joes

Time: 30 Minutes

Servings: 6

Ingredients:

- Whole Grain Buns (12 halves)
- Vegan Worcestershire Sauce (1 T.)
- Ketchup (.25 C.)
- Tomato Puree (1 Can)
- Cooked Wheat Berries (2 C.)
- Minced Garlic (2)
- Chopped Green Bell Pepper (.50 C.)
- Chopped Celery (.50 C.)
- Chopped Onion (.50 C.)
- Pitted Dates (.33 C.)

Directions:

1. To start this recipe, first, place one third of a cup of water and dates into a pot and cook over a medium to low heat for around 10 minutes. By the end, the dates should be soft and tender so you can quickly pop them into your blender to puree until they become nice and creamy.

2. After that, you will want to place the bell pepper, celery, and onion into the skillet and cook over a

medium heat for 8 minutes. Once they are cooked, add in the garlic, cooked wheat berries, date paste, tomato puree, Worcestershire sauce, and ketchup. Go ahead and cook everything for 10 more minutes or until the mixture becomes thick.

3. Finally, slather a generous amount of the mixture in between two buns and enjoy warm!

4. Quinoa and Hummus Wraps

Time: 15 Minutes

Servings: 4

Ingredients:

- Whole Wheat Tortillas (4)
- Sliced Tomatoes (2)
- Fresh Spinach (2 C.)
- Cooked Quinoa (1 C.)
- Hummus (2 C.)

Directions:

1. This recipe is perfect if you need a quick and easy dinner. To start out, you're going to want to lay out your tortillas.
2. Once this is done, spread the hummus evenly across the tortilla and then place the cooked quinoa on top of that.
3. Top it off with the spinach and tomato, then roll up the tortillas and dinner is served!

Kick-start Your Plant-Based Lifestyle

5. Chickpea Burgers

Time: 50 Minutes

Servings: 8

Ingredients:

- Whole Grain Buns (16 halves)
- Rolled Oats (1 C.)
- Fresh Thyme (1 t.)
- Black Pepper (.10 t.)
- Dijon Mustard (.50 t.)
- Red Wine Vinegar (1 t.)
- Salt (.10 t.)
- Tomato Paste (1 T.)
- Nutritional Yeast (.50 C.)
- Chickpeas (2 Cans)
- Garlic (1)
- Chopped Red Bell Pepper (.50 C.)
- Sliced Carrots (1 C.)
- Romaine lettuce (Optional)
- Sliced Tomatoes (Optional)

Directions:

1. To start these delicious burgers, you will first have to get your food processor out. Then, add in the garlic, bell pepper, and carrots. Go ahead and pulse

Kick-start Your Plant-Based Lifestyle

these ingredients until they are all finely chopped.

2. Once this first step is completed, add in the rest of the ingredients minus your rolled oats, whole grain buns and the optional lettuce and tomatoes. If needed, scrape down the sides of your food processor and continue to blend until everything is smooth. Once smooth, you can now add in the rolled oats and pulse again for about 5 to 7 times.

3. Next, you will want to place the mixture into the fridge for 30 minutes to allow it to settle.

4. When you are ready, take it out from the fridge and scoop the mixture with your hands and begin to make patties. This should make 7 or 8 patties, depending on the size.

5. Finally, heat up a skillet and cook the patties on either side for 8 minutes. You will know they're cooked when they're golden-brown on both sides.

6. Finally, assemble your burgers. You can add some lettuce or tomatoes if you like, and enjoy your plant-based dinner!

Kick-start Your Plant-Based Lifestyle

Your Meal Plan:

	Sun	Mon	Tue	Wed	Thurs	Fri	Sat
Breakfast		Overnight Oats	Stuffed Sweet Potato	Overnight Oats	Plant-based Breakfast Burritos	Black Bean and Corn Cake	Oat Waffles
Lunch		Red Pepper and Tomato Soup	Left-over Sloppy Joes	Stuffed Lettuce Cups	White Bean and Cauliflower Soup	Left-over Mac and Cheese	Left-over White Bean and Cauliflower Soup
Dinner		Sloppy Joes	Lemon Dijon Cauliflower	Quinoa and Hummus Wraps	Mac and Cheese	Chickpea Burgers	Lemon Dijon Cauliflower

Kick-start Your Plant-Based Lifestyle

Plant-based Grocery List

Vegetables

- o Red and Green Bell Peppers
- o Jalapeno Peppers
- o Green Chilies
- o Fresh Parsley
- o Carrots
- o Scallions
- o Garlic
- o Green onions
- o Onions
- o Sweet Potatoes
- o Potatoes
- o Romaine Lettuce Hearts
- o Leeks
- o Cauliflower
- o Corn or Frozen corn kernels
- o Carrots
- o Green Beans
- o Spinach
- o Cilantro
- o Brussel Sprouts
- o Eggplant
- o Swiss Chard

Kick-start Your Plant-Based Lifestyle

- Sprouted Greens
- Watercress
- Salad Greens
- Butternut Squash
- Pumpkin
- Zucchini
- Beets
- Radishes
- Celery
- Parsnips
- Asparagus
- Broccoli
- Collard Greens
- Kale

Fruits

- Regular and Cherry Tomatoes
- Mangoes
- Limes
- Lemons
- Oranges
- Raspberries
- Blackberries
- Cranberries
- Blueberries
- Bananas

Kick-start Your Plant-Based Lifestyle

- Dates
- Pomegranate
- Papaya
- Figs
- Kiwi
- Watermelon
- Avocado
- Melons
- Bananas
- Nectarines
- Coconut
- Mulberries
- Plums
- Cherries
- Peaches
- Passion Fruit

Raw and Unsalted Nuts & Seeds

- Hemp Seeds
- Ground Flaxseeds
- Sunflower Seeds
- Sesame Seeds
- Chia Seeds
- Quinoa
- Almond Butter
- Almonds

Kick-start Your Plant-Based Lifestyle

- Cashews
- Pistachios
- Hazelnuts
- Brazil Nuts
- Pine Nuts
- Walnuts
- Pecans
- Pumpkin Seeds

Legumes

- Chickpeas
- Black Beans
- Pinto Beans
- Cannellini White Beans
- Lime Beans
- Kidney Beans
- Black-eyed Peas
- Snow Peas
- Split Peas
- Snap Peas
- Green Peas
- Lentils (black, green, yellow, red)

Spices & Condiments

Kick-start Your Plant-Based Lifestyle

- Cinnamon
- Salt
- Black Pepper
- Chili Powder
- Hot Sauce
- Red Pepper Flakes
- Fresh & Dried Thyme
- Rosemary
- Ground Turmeric
- Dried Basil
- Fresh Oregano
- Hummus
- Dijon Mustard
- Ketchup
- Tomato Puree
- Tomato Paste
- Pure Maple Syrup
- Vegan Worcestershire Sauce
- Unsweetened Applesauce

Whole Grains

- Wheat Berries
- Whole Grain Penne
- Whole Grain Buns
- Whole Wheat Tortilla Wraps
- Rolled Oats

Kick-start Your Plant-Based Lifestyle

- Whole Wheat Pastry Flour
- Cornmeal
- Sorghum
- Buckwheat
- Amaranth
- Brown Rice
- Millet

Others

- Vanilla Extract
- Extra firm Tofu
- Nutritional Yeast
- Unsweetened Plant Milk (either Soy or Almond)
- White Wine Vinegar
- Red Wine Vinegar
- White Miso Paste
- Baking Powder

Kick-start Your Plant-Based Lifestyle

As you can probably tell, this is an expandable grocery list, but for now it's good enough to help you get started. As you go along your plant-based diet journey, you'll be able to tell which foods you can enjoy and which you should probably avoid. In case you're still unsure, in the next chapter, I'll provide you with more tips and tricks for the plant-based diet.

Chapter Seven:
Tips and Tricks for Real Life

Switching over to a new diet can be very intimidating, especially if you are just starting out. If you're anything like me, I know you've either been eating the same unhealthy way all your life, or you have been bouncing from diet to diet searching for answers. I hope I've provided enough value to you so far such that you're convinced that the plant-based diet is truly beneficial for you and your loved ones! However, I love to provide you with even more value. Thus, to ensure you really feel comfortable moving forward, I've included some of my favorite tips to help you get started and stay motivated!

Believe in Yourself

Although there are many misconceptions about the plant-based diet, do not let them distract you. Believe in your food choices and just keep going, slowly you'll find that the plant-based lifestyle will become more and more abundant in your life. Even on your first trip to the grocery store on a plant-based diet, you'll begin to notice all the vegan products available.

I am a true believer that 80% of any success story is having the right mindset. A big part of this mindset is having self-belief and to fully trust the process! Self-belief will also guide you in making decisions that are aligned with your goals. To help you get into this winning mindset, I just want to remind you that you're already way ahead of the pack because you have this book of knowledge. That's an incredible advantage for you to take back control of your life.

Take Small Bites

I mean this literally and figuratively. Nobody is expecting you to change your diet cold turkey. I don't want you to wake up tomorrow morning and tell yourself, "no more animal products forever!" Unfortunately, this will only cause you to panic and binge. Instead, I suggest you give up one item at a time. Perhaps to begin, try eating a plant-based meal once or twice a week. As you become more comfortable with this new way of eating, you can then take the next step of replacing more food items in your diet.

At the beginning, when you're trying to reduce consumption of meat, it's very normal to fall back into your old eating habits. If that happens, you can help yourself by reducing the amount of meat you are eating in a week instead of in a day. The same goes for dairy and egg products. When you take smaller steps, it not raises your chance of following through; it also boosts your confidence as you make these small wins along the way. As time goes on, you'd be surprised to learn that everything feels much easier.

Say Goodbye to Labels

For some reason, we feel the need to label everything and everyone. You'll get many people trying to put you in a box by calling you a vegan or vegetarian and segregating you from the others based on your diet choice. You might feel left out sometimes. However, do not mind them. Let people label you however way they want. As long as you stay strong and do not let it deter you from staying on your plant-based diet, you're on your way to a healthier and happier life. In the end, trying is better than not attempting at all!

As you begin to make healthier food choices, it's

normal to slip up. I don't want you to go into this lifestyle expecting to be perfect. Focus on progress instead of perfection. Don't label yourself as well because that's putting too much pressure on you. If you become too strict on yourself, your brain will push back and trick you into craving for those exact items you were trying to cut back on. I suggest you learn to not stress over the little things. As long as you're consistent, you will begin to see the changes. Instead of beating yourself up, move on and carry on with your healthy lifestyle. One slip up won't ruin all of your hard work, I promise.

Follow Your Budget

In Chapter 2, we learnt that a plant-based diet isn't as expensive as most people think it is, but I imagine you will still have a budget when it comes to grocery shopping. As you go through the store, try to be conscious of where you're spending your money. I suggest you shop the perimeter of the store, as this is where most plant-based foods are going to be. Stick with fresh produce as much as possible, but frozen foods are always a great alternative! Beware of the center aisles as they are typically packed with processed foods. If it's summer, give your farmer's market a visit and support your local food providers. It is a win-win for everyone involved, including the planet!

Remember Your Why

This is very important! In the beginning of any diet, it is very easy to get super pumped up and excited. However, it is normal for people lose steam along the way. As I've mentioned earlier, a plant-based diet is going to take consistent work. This diet will slowly change into a lifestyle and require you to put in the time and effort day in and day out. So you must continually remind yourself of your "why" and pump yourself up on bad days. Any time you catch yourself slipping just remember why you got started in the first place and it would put you back on track.

Learn to Speak Up

A majority of people does not follow a plant-based diet. In fact, you should go into this journey prepared for eye-rolls and questions from your friends and family. You will probably find this lifestyle even more challenging when you go out to a restaurant. My tip for you is to learn to speak up! You would be surprised to learn just how accommodating restaurants can be or how flexible an item on the menu can become. Of course, I'm not suggesting that you should demand everyone to go above and beyond for your needs, but it doesn't hurt to ask. If all else fails, you can't go wrong with a big salad!

Dining Out

I want you to take a minute and try to answer these 2 questions. First, "how many fast food restaurants are near to your house right now?" And second, "how many times a week do you eat at these fast food joints?" Bearing your answers in mind, one of the most important things I want you to try to do is limit your visits to these fast food joints as you begin a plant-based diet.

However, if you are invited out for dinner to a fast food joint or any place where they do not serve any plant-based food at all, the best thing to do is propose an alternative. If that is not possible, simply reject the invitation. Most people say yes to invitations like this out of guilt or the need to please. You should not feel bad if you say "no". However, saying no also requires some grace. Here's a way of rejecting your friends or family without sounding rude – you can say, "thank you for your invite but I'll give it a miss, while it is not something that agrees with my eating habits, please know how grateful I am to be asked." If you face any pushbacks, do not cave. Simply remember your why and stay firm. You could reply them by saying this – "I'd just rather not but thank you for thinking of me."

Learn to Cook

The easiest and most hassle-free option is definitely to cook your own meals. Therefore, it is vital that you brush up on your cooking skills.

For this reason, I've provided you with those delicious recipes in Chapter 6, for breakfast, lunch, and dinner to help you get started! A plant-based diet is completely doable, but if you're new to cooking, I suggest that you learn how to cook first. Your food will only taste as good as your ability to prepare them. With a solid cooking foundation, you'll be addicted to whipping up those amazing plant-based delicacies!

Stock Up

If you are looking to set yourself up for success, having a properly stocked pantry is going to be very important. Before you even begin, I suggest getting rid of any processed foods you have. By doing this, you will be getting rid of any temptations. Instead of the Cheetos and Oreos, it is time to stock your pantry with delicious plant-based whole foods.

I find that the best way to go about this is to stay

organized! Before you do your grocery shopping, try to get your meal plan together. In the chapter before, I've provided you with a grocery list and a sample meal plan. While this is meant to be a jumping off point, I suggest you start creating a habit of planning your meals every week. This way, you'll be able to get what you need on your grocery runs while keeping your pantry properly stocked!

Support Each Other

When I first started a plant-based diet, only a small group of people supported me. The rest would try to get me to eat ice cream or a double-cheese beef-burger and tell me that I was being ridiculous from "denying" myself these delicious foods. It was hard to be polite and explain to them that I was doing this for my own health and my family's as well. Instead of getting angry and defensive, kindly ask for support instead. If not, there is always an online forum or a Facebook group for you to be a part of. There're plenty of people out there who are going through the same diet and are facing the same challenges as you. When you begin anything in life, a support system is always a great way to stay motivated.

Learn to Read

Kick-start Your Plant-Based Lifestyle

You know very well by this point that processed foods are going to be a big no-no on a plant-based diet. It will be important to become a master at reading the labels on your food. You may be shocked to learn just how many items contain animal products; this includes your drinks as well! Instead of buying food in packages, I suggest sticking to fresh and whole foods. If a food doesn't have a label, it is most likely whole. Stick with them instead, and you'll be safe.

Learn to Love Vegetables

From now on, vegetables are going to be the star of your meal. Up until now, your vegetables have most likely just been a side dish, but now I want them to take up a majority of your plate. Luckily, veggies come in different colors and flavors, so you'll never be bored. Build a curiosity and love for trying all sorts of vegetables out there because they will provide you with a variety of nutrients that are good for you. If you are struggling to find a vegetable that you truly enjoy, take a few minutes to look at the grocery list provided to you in the previous chapter. I assure you that there is at least one vegetable for every person in your family.

Keep an Open Mind

There might come a time where you'll hit a plateau. There are going to be nights where you don't feel like cooking and get tempted to just order pizza instead, and that is perfectly understandable. When that happens, I invite you to take a deep breath and remember why you started this journey in the first place.

Then, open up your mind and reflect on how the benefits are already reflecting in your quality of life. You've started to sleep more soundly, you've begun losing weight and are feeling more energized. Any time you lose motivation, simply remind yourself of all these benefits you're manifesting in your life. Keep an open mind that more of them will come your way if you just keep putting in the work.

We are finally moving into the final chapter! Here, I'll be giving you my 3 personal secrets to success. Remember, a plant-based diet is so much more than just the foods you are going to enjoy. It is also about living healthier and happier. When you're willing to put in the work, you will experience incredible results.

Chapter Eight:
The Secret to Success

While general tips and tricks are important, I'm also here to tell you 3 proven-to-work secrets that I've used for myself when I was transitioning to a plant-based diet. This is as far as I can go to provide you the best value to attain success. Ultimately, you have to remember what is important here; YOU! You are worth it, and you are going to work hard for yourself because nobody else can do that for you.

#1 Secret: Meal Prep for Success

If you're looking to save time and money, meal prepping is going to be a lifesaver for you! Coming up, I'll

Kick-start Your Plant-Based Lifestyle

be sharing some of my favorite tips that will make meal prepping a breeze, even if you're a beginner. Meal prep is literally a cheat-code to setting yourself up for success. Once you've got it nailed down, there will be very little room to fail.

1. Make Your Plan

Sit down and pull out a food journal. I want you to take a few minutes to write a list of your favorite healthy foods. Once you have this list, use the Internet to find simple recipes containing foods on your list. Then choose the ones that allow you to cook in bulk and in a timely fashion.

There is no such thing as over-prepping when it comes to meal prep. If you can, try to plan for every meal and every snack. I promise that as you do this weekly, you will get better at it. To make it easier, you can use the meal plan provided in the chapter 6 as a reference. To save even more time, compile all your meal plans from each week in your food journal, so they are easily accessible and can be recycled again at some point. Once you've a few menus created, you can rotate them to keep your diet fun and exciting!

2. Only Buy From Your List

Once you have your recipes, you will want to

create a grocery list. With a list, it will be easier to go to the store and grab only what you need. This means, there won't be room for junk food in your cart because it's not on the list. As you work on your self-belief, your willpower will become strong enough to avoid the temptations of foods you don't need. However, meanwhile, a grocery list is the best way to ensure that you only buy the good stuff and ignore your bad impulse. Also, when you avoid impulse buys, you're actually saving money too!

3. Short Cuts

Figure out little shortcuts that can quickly get the cooking done and help you get onto the fun part; eating! For myself, I like to buy pre-cut fruits and vegetables, so that cutting them up isn't another step I have to take before cooking or using them in my recipes. As I've hinted in chapter 2, these pre-cut fruits and vegetables are my top choice to have on hand as snacks. I like to keep them packed nicely in small storage containers so they are easily accessible and I stop myself from reaching for junk food or start calling pizza delivery. The goal here is to find ways to make your plant-based diet more convenient.

4. Food Storage Containers

If you're serious about meal prepping, then I

highly suggest you invest in food containers. When you're deciding on what to buy, go for a variety of sizes so you can cover all types of meals – from mains to side dishes to snacks. You will also want to make sure that the containers are microwave-safe, dishwasher-safe, and BPA-free. This way, you will be able to keep your whole foods fresher, longer and heat them up easily when needed. Just remember that fresh foods expire quicker than processed foods, but having containers can help to slightly prolong it.

5. Mix It Up

Look up recipes beforehand so you'll always have an inventory of new recipes to try out. You'd be amazed at how many delicious and easy plant-based recipes are out there on the Internet. There are incredible blogs and books dedicated to recipes that are innovative and delicious.

In fact, later on in this bundle, you'll have full access to my plant-based cookbook, which I've published just a few months ago. Inside it, you will find 15 Quick & Easy Plant-based Recipes for Weight Loss & Nutrition.

If you are a fan of cooking and love trying out new recipes, you'll never run out of the variety that goes into your new plant-based lifestyle!

#2 Secret: Exercise and a Plant-based Diet

While a plant-based diet is going to be important for your health, this is much more about living a healthier lifestyle to benefit the most from your food choices. There are many incredible benefits from exercising, and you don't have to run a marathon to gain these benefits. Now, I will share some of these benefits and help you get started on a new exercise regimen.

1. Helps Prevent Disease

Our bodies are meant to move! If you wish to have good physical fitness and health, regular exercise is going to be very important on a regular basis. Studies have shown that regular exercise may improve insulin sensitivity. On the other hand, a study published in the research journal called "Obesity" showed that a lack of exercise could increase the risk of heart disease and type 2 diabetes. What this means is that eating better is essential but regular exercise will add an extra layer of defense for you.

2. Energy Levels

Studies have shown that exercise acts as one of the best energy boosters for people. There was one particular study done on 36 healthy people who reported frequent bouts of fatigue. After just 6 short weeks of putting them on a regular exercise regimen, they reported reduced feelings of fatigue. It seems like exercise really has the ability to increase energy levels for those who have chronic fatigue syndrome.

3. Weight Loss

While eating a healthy, plant-based diet will help you lose weight, a Finland study from its National Public Health Institute has shown that one of the major contributors to obesity and weight gain is inactivity. In order to understand this, you must first understand that there is a direct relationship between energy expenditure and exercise.

You see, your body maintains bodily functions; these activities require energy. When you begin to diet, you will be reducing your caloric intake, which will lower your metabolic rate. When this happens, it could delay the weight loss you are seeking. With this in mind, regular exercise has the ability to increase your metabolic rate and burn more calories without delaying your weight loss. By exercising, you'll also be able to maintain your weight loss and grow muscle mass!

4. It Makes You Happier

If you're looking to improve your mood, decrease stress,

anxiety, and depression, then exercise is going to be your new best friend! Studies have shown that when we exercise, the part of our brain that regulates anxiety and stress changes. Through exercise, we increase the sensitivity of our brain to hormones including norepinephrine and serotonin, which helps relieve the feelings of depression.

The best part is that it doesn't seem to matter how intense your workout is. You can improve your mood no matter what kind of physical activity you choose to do. Later on, I'll provide you with more information on the 3 ways to move your body.

5. Brain Health

How many of us walk into a room and completely forget why we were there in the first place? Luckily, exercise can help to protect our memories, build thinking skills and improve our rain function! From a scientific standpoint, this may be due to the fact that exercise increases the heart rate and in turn, promotes the flow of oxygen and blood in the brain. Exercise also stimulates the growth of hormones and brain cells.

Studies have shown that through regular physical activity, older adults are able to change and enhance the function and structure of their brain. In fact, exercise can grow the hippocampus, which is vital for learning and memories. In a study published in the Current Alzheimer Research journal, it was found that exercise could help to reduce changes in the brain that eventually lead to Alzheimer's disease, as well as schizophrenia in some individuals.

6. Reduce Pain

Many people who deal with chronic illnesses also have chronic pain. Unfortunately, this pain can be incredibly debilitating for our daily tasks. While for so many years, doctors have suggested inactivity to deal with the pain, recent studies have shown that exercise can help relieve this pain! In particular, regular exercise seems to benefit chronic soft tissue shoulder disorder and chronic lower back pain among others.

The bottom line is that regular physical activity combined with healthy and whole foods can help you both internally and externally to improve nearly every aspect of your health. Now, I'll help get you started with some simple exercise regiments.

Common Exercises

- Strength

Strength building will help you to increase the strength and power of your muscles. Some popular examples include weight lifting, resistance training, and plyometrics like jumping rope or jump squats.

- Aerobic

Aerobics are typically the core of any fitness program that you decide to follow. Some of the more popular aerobic exercises include dancing, running, hiking and swimming.

- Calisthenics

This is a type of exercise involving basic body movements that you can perform at home, without the use of any gym equipment. Some popular examples would be pull-ups, push-ups, sit-ups, and lunges!

How Much Exercise?

There is no need to become a high-performance athlete overnight! According to the American College of Sports Medicine, there is a recommendation of 150 minutes of aerobic exercise per week. This can be broken down in a number of different ways whether you want to do 40-minutes workouts every other day or 30-minutes workouts 5 times a week. It all depends on your schedule and what works best for you. At the end of the day, as long as you are engaging in physical activity regularly, you'll be benefiting your health!

I think it's also important to note that resting is just as crucial as working out. If you do not allow your body enough time to recover from a hard workout session, it could lead to muscle strains and stress fractures. On top of this, too much exercise might weaken your immune system and increase the risk of chronic fatigue, depression, hormonal imbalances and infection. Instead, try to start out slow and constantly adjust according to your limits.

#3 Secret: Healthy Affirmations

Along with your healthy lifestyle, you will want to keep your mental health in mind. When your mind has the ability to think healthy thoughts, your body will find it easier to be healthy because there is a connection between the body and mind. On the flipside, you can also see how your thoughts and emotions might cause disruption to your health if you think disempowering thoughts.

Once you've learnt how to change your thoughts, you will change your life. Through positive and healthy affirmations, you're actually promoting health to yourself so that both the health of your body and the health of your mind are aligned. I understand that starting a new lifestyle can be difficult and scary, but these affirmations can help to make the transition much smoother.

Now, I'm going to share with you 10 of my favorite affirmations to get through the trying times.

1. I choose to make healthy choices every single day.
2. I avoid eating junk food; I only consume healthy plant-based foods because I respect my body and only provide it with the best.
3. I am in perfect health because I take care of my body.
4. Each and every cell in my body is healed and full of life.
5. It does not matter what the external conditions are, I'm always grateful for my health.
6. I choose to have positive energy; I only focus on being happy and I release all the ill feelings I've felt before.
7. I am energetic and full of vitality because I'm fueled by plant foods.
8. I am calm, relaxed and have great coping skills.
9. I love myself as I am; I am confident of how I look.
10. I enjoy eating healthy and living a plant-based lifestyle. I am in this for the long haul.

Conclusion

We have reached the final lap of this book. I hope that you're feeling excited to start your new lifestyle! If at any point in time, you start to have self-doubts on any aspect of the plant-based diet, I invite you to re-visit that particular section of this book for a touch-up on your knowledge. Really immerse yourself and apply the knowledge in your real life. There're so many incredible benefits for you to experience; I truly only want the best for anyone looking to better their health.

As I've mentioned, I was not only able to change my own life, I saw firsthand how it has improved my boys' lives too. It is wonderful to know that we are choosing the plant-based lifestyle not only for ourselves but also for the one planet we have been gifted with. It is up to us to improve our health and save our environment because nobody else is going to do it for us! I hope we can all band together and create a new ray of hope for future generations.

Lastly, I wish you the best of luck on your new plant-based journey. Go out there and enjoy it!

I choose to recognize that my past is behind me.

*Now, I choose to be present and
will decide my own Destiny.*

I have many opportunities, and my options are plentiful.

I choose to eat plant-based to benefit not only me

but also this beautiful planet earth, which I live on.

I am healthy.

I am happy.

I am whole.

Kick-start Your Plant-Based Lifestyle

Kick-start Your Plant-Based Lifestyle

Plant-Based Diet

A Beginner's Cookbook - 15 Quick & Easy Plant-based Recipes for Weight Loss & Nutrition

By: Alyani Cook

Kick-start Your Plant-Based Lifestyle

Foreword

I would like to dedicate this Cookbook to my grandmother.

For being so wise.
For shining the light on me on my darkest days.
For loving me as I am.

I can see her smiling at me, saying,
"You are the heart of my heart, Aly."

I love you Nana.

What is a Plant-based Diet?

An Introduction

Just a few months ago, I was severely overweight and in really bad shape. I am a stay-at-home mom. I am a proud mother of 2 lovely and intelligent sons. Unfortunately, my health was beginning to get in the way of being the mother that I know I can be. I just felt so terrible that I could not do what seems so easy for any other mothers out there.

I couldn't go out to play with them during the weekends because I was so embarrassed by my appearance. I couldn't sleep well and would feel so lethargic the following day. I honestly felt like I was the biggest let down in their lives.

Then, one weekend, while my 2 boys were once again stuck at home because their mom was too sick to bring them out, I decided to make a change. I did not know how to make what change but I had a computer, I knew how to google and I was desperate. Indeed, I was so desperate I typed into Google: "best diets".

After scrolling around for a few minutes, I closed my eyes and randomly picked one. Believe it or not, yes, I picked the plant-based diet.

I am not trying to be dramatic here but I must say stumbling onto the plant-based diet has definitely changed my life completely.

The change was not just for my own health. It also improved the overall well-being of my boys and my friends and family. I shed the weight so easily I could not believe it. I started sharing the plant-based diet with my neighbors and the other moms at the park. I must say my social life improved dramatically as well, after I finally gained enough confidence to leave the house with my boys.

Everything was looking up.

Then one day, while I was looking for more interesting things to share about the plant-based diet, I chanced upon a study about how eating a plant-based diet not only affects our health, it also affects our planet.

In fact, it can lower global emissions by a whooping 75%! I am no expert on the health of our planet but I know 75% is a huge drop and will make a significant difference.

That was when eating plant based became a mission, it became bigger than me. Look, I am a mom with 2 boys that I love so much. My biggest wish is for them to live in a beautiful world. A world that is free from pollution and disease.

So now, I am publishing a cookbook with quick and easy delicious recipes that I have created. This is a gift from my heart because I believe we can all do better for our children.

What is a Plant Based Diet?

A plant-based diet is one that relies on the various plants that Mother Nature produces. As the name implies, there are little to no animal products in a plant-based diet. In general, there are two levels of "plant-based" eating you can follow.

If you still want to consume certain dairy products

and ingredients such as honey, which are produced by animals, you would want to follow a vegetarian eating plan. This allows you to continue consuming milk, cheeses, and similar products, which can allow for more flexibility.

However, many other people who follow a plant-based diet do not believe in consuming any animal products whatsoever. If you are one of them, that would put you into the vegan category, which have been proven to be much healthier by experts in the nutrition field.

Animal by-products, like milk, can contain hormones, bacteria, and other compounds that some research suggests could harm your health. Dairy products are also linked to skin conditions, like acne, so there are many valid reasons to try and avoid it.

In addition to bringing more health and nutritional benefits, a plant-based diet also helps with weight loss. Why? Because it is naturally more fiber-rich!

The magic about fiber is that it keeps you full. You are less likely to feel hungry and go off snacking throughout the day. And so, chances of you putting on weight is much lower. In fact, you will start to shed off the extra pounds from all those unnecessary snacking, and keep the weight off for a longer time.

Kick-start Your Plant-Based Lifestyle

Regardless of your motivation, though, there are some myths that you should see debunked before diving further into the world of plant-based eating.

Where will I get my protein?

Meat is far from the only protein source out there. If you are going to follow a vegetarian diet, then you can continue drinking milk or using whey protein (a derivative of milk). Dairy milk is a complete protein, which means it contains all nine essential amino acids.

But, if you want to limit dairy, you're in luck. There are actually many plant-based complete proteins that will also give your body all nine essential amino acids. This includes buckwheat, quinoa, and soy protein. Many other plants also contain protein, but they are not considered "complete" proteins because they don't contain all nine essential amino acids.

Will I be able to afford a plant-based diet?

It's a fact: junk food like chips and soda is cheap. Often, it seems substantially cheaper than healthy foods like fruits and veggies. But, when you begin to look at the bigger picture, you'll start to see how much junk food will cost you.

Kick-start Your Plant-Based Lifestyle

Junk food will negatively impact your health in the long-term. And, in the short-term, it's going to cost you in the form of bigger servings. Junk food will never satisfy your hunger and it often leads to over-eating. Chips and soda is nothing more than "empty" calories that do not fill you up and provide no nutritional value.

So, eating a plant-based diet means eating real, whole foods that provide your body with the nutrition it needs while being filling and flavorful.

Challenge Yourself!

Have you ever bought a cookbook just to have it sit on the shelf collecting dust? Don't let that be this book! After you have spent some time drooling over the recipes, make a plan. Get out your calendar and mark down some dates where you'll try these recipes. They're made using seasonal ingredients which will save you money and lead to the best flavor!

Once you've made each recipe by the book, try putting your own unique spin on it. The kitchen is a great place to let your creativity shine! With your twist added, post a picture of it on Instagram with the #PlantBasedDietChallenge.

Now, let's dive in!

In The Spring

In the springtime, lots of plants are coming into bloom. Here's a look at some of the fantastic ingredients to look for:

- Arugula: High in Vitamin A, Vitamin K, and folate, Arugula has lots of benefits. It even provides fiber, chlorophyll, and lots of water! That can keep you hydrated while detoxifying your body and reducing inflammation.

- Artichokes: Also rich in folic acid, artichoke contains Vitamin C and B-complex vitamins along with lots of minerals. Lower your cholesterol and reduce free radicals with this green food.

- Asparagus: Lots of Vitamin K will help prevent cancer and boost heart and bone health. Copper, selenium, and B vitamins and other vitamins to improve your well-being.

- Strawberries: One of the top five most antioxidant rich fruits in the United States, strawberries are a decadent fruit that can balance your blood sugar and support your immunity.

Sliced Artichoke and Baby Arugula Salad

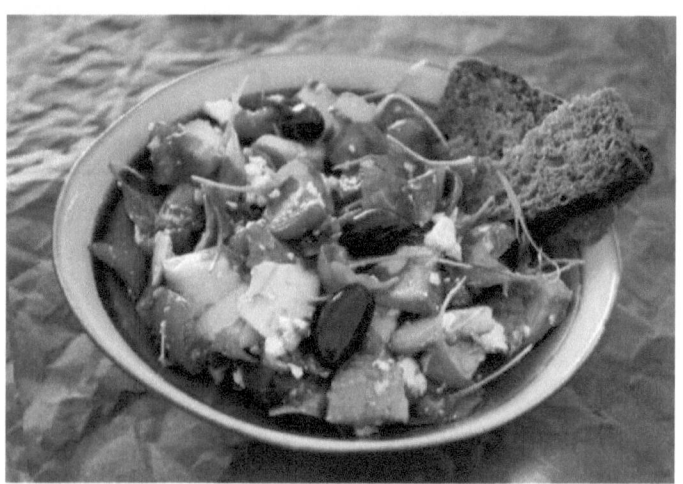

Ingredients

- 8 cups baby arugula leaves
- 8 oil-packed artichoke hearts, drained, patted dry, and cut in 1/4-inch slices
- 1/4 cup sliced pitted kalamata olives, optional
- 2 cups grape tomatoes, halved
- 4 tablespoons chopped fresh chives
- 3 Tbs. olive oil
- 1 Tbs. aged balsamic vinegar
- 2 cloves garlic, minced (2 tsp.)

Kick-start Your Plant-Based Lifestyle

Directions

1. Make the Vinaigrette by whisking the olive oil and balsamic vinegar together in a small bowl. Add salt and pepper to taste.
2. To make the salad, toss everything together and top off with tomatoes and chives. Season with black pepper to taste. Add vinaigrette and serve!

Creamy Vegan Lemon Asparagus Pasta

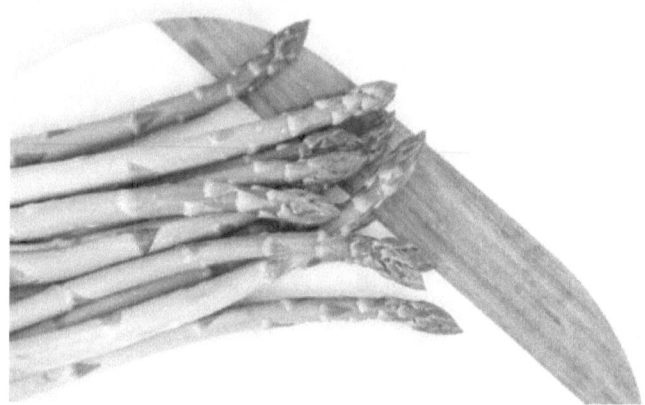

Ingredients

- 1 bunch asparagus, trimmed and washed
- 2 medium lemons, sliced thinly
- Juice of half a lemon
- 3 1/2 tablespoons olive oil, divided
- 3-4 large cloves garlic, minced
- 5 cups bow tie pasta (10 ounces)
- 2 1/2 cups unsweetened plain almond milk
- 3-4 tablespoons all-purpose flour
- Salt and black pepper

Directions

Kick-start Your Plant-Based Lifestyle

1. Preheat the oven to 400 degrees F.
2. In a baking sheet, toss asparagus and half a tablespoon of olive oil with a pinch of salt and pepper. Top with thin slices of lemon and bake for 25 minutes. Chop into thirds when finished cooking.
3. Bring a pot of water to a boil and add salt.
4. Bring a large skillet to medium heat then add three tablespoons of olive oil and garlic. Whisk and cook for 1-2 minutes so garlic browns. Add three tablespoons of flour and cook for 30 seconds. Whisk in almond milk a half cup at a time. Add salt and pepper then whisk. Lower heat slightly and continue stirring until thickened.
5. Boil the pasta and cook based on the package's directions. Drain and set aside.
6. If sauce is runny, add remaining flour. Add the juice of half a lemon and stir. Add the pasta and 3/4 of the chopped asparagus then toss to coat.
7. Serve and enjoy!

Raw Strawberry Cheesecake

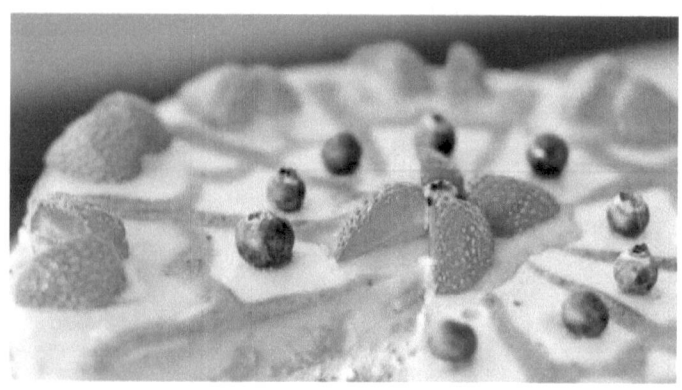

Ingredients

- 2 cups raw cashews, soaked overnight and drained
- 2 cups strawberries, plus more for decoration
- 1 cup raw pecans
- 1 cup dates, divided
- ½ cup rolled oats
- 1 tablespoon maple syrup
- ½ teaspoon sea salt
- ¼ teaspoon cinnamon
- Blueberries for decoration

Directions

Kick-start Your Plant-Based Lifestyle

1. If you use small, dry, and hard dates, soak them for about 15 minutes in hot water. If you use large and soft dates, you do not need to soak them.
2. In a food processor, combine pecans, oats, salt, cinnamon, and a half cup of the dates. Blend until soft and grainy. Press into the bottom of a pie pan.
3. Now place strawberries, cashews, remaining dates, and maple syrup into the food processor. Blend until smooth. Pour the mixture over the crust, decorating the top with strawberries and blueberries.
4. Freeze for three or more hours and enjoy!

In The Summer

The summertime is filled with delicious ingredients that are colorful and flavorful, including:

- Apricots: A great source of fiber and Vitamin A, apricots are good for your heart, blood, and skin thanks to a variety of antioxidants.

- Plums: Containing fiber, antioxidants, vitamins, and minerals of all kinds, plums reduce the risk of heart disease and diabetes.

- Cherries: Filled with antioxidants and anti-inflammatory compounds, cherries can help you sleep better while reducing joint pain and speeding up recovery from exercise.

- Tomatoes: With Lycopene and other antioxidants, tomatoes reduce the risk of heart disease and cancer. They also contain Vitamin C, Vitamin K, potassium, and folate.

Apricot Muffins

Baking is a great way to escape the heat and get indoors. Plus, these refreshing muffins add a sweet but light and bright start to anyone's day.

(no photo for this recipe.)

Ingredients

- 1 tablespoon chia seed meal mixed with 3 tablespoons of water
- 1 1/2 cups whole wheat flour
- 1/2 cup all-purpose flour
- 1 1/2 teaspoons baking powder
- 1 teaspoon baking soda
- 1/2 teaspoon sea salt
- 1 teaspoon ground cinnamon
- 1/2 cup brown rice syrup
- 1/4 cup maple syrup
- 3/4 cup plus 2 tablespoons almond milk
- 1/4 cup olive oil
- 1 cup apricots dried and pulsed in food processor
- 1/2 cup almonds finely chopped in a food processor

Kick-start Your Plant-Based Lifestyle

Directions

1. Preheat your oven to 425 degrees F.
2. Lightly oil a muffin tin for 12 muffins.
3. Mix egg replacer and water and set aside.
4. In a large bowl, combine the flours with the cinnamon, baking powder, baking soda, and salt.
5. Add the syrups, milk, and oil to the dry mixture then stir just to combine. Fold in the apricot and almonds.
6. Bake for 15 to 20 minutes until baked through.
7. Allow to cool for 10 minutes.

Spiced Plum Crumble

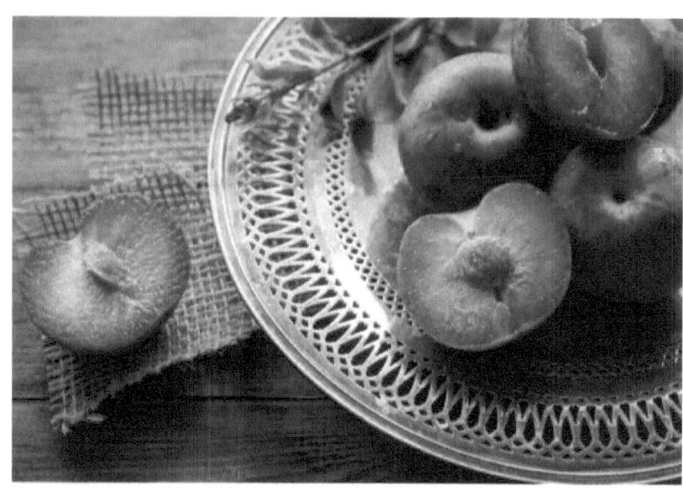

Crumb Ingredients:

- 2 cups of all-purpose flour
- 4½ oz of vegan butter
- ½ cup of demerara sugar
- ⅛ cup of white sugar
- 2 ounces of ground almonds
- 2 tbsp slivered almonds
- pinch of sea salt

Filling Ingredients:

- 2 lbs of fresh plums, stones removed

Kick-start Your Plant-Based Lifestyle

- 2 tbsp demerara sugar
- 1 vanilla pod, seeds only
- 1 tsp ground cinnamon
- ½ tsp ground anise
- ½ tsp ground nutmeg
- pinch ground cloves
- pinch ground cardamom

Directions:

1. Preheat your oven to 400 degrees F.
2. Combine the flour, salt, and butter into a food processor. Pulse until the mixture resembles breadcrumbs then add the demerara sugar and white sugar. Add ground almonds and pulse to mix.
3. Place the plums into a mixing bowl and the remaining ingredients for the filling. Mix to coat the plums with all the spices.
4. Arrange the plums in a deep pie pan and then spread the crumble coating on the top. Sprinkle with slivered almonds.
5. Bake for about 35 minutes until golden brown. Let rest 10 minutes before serving.

Cherry Delight

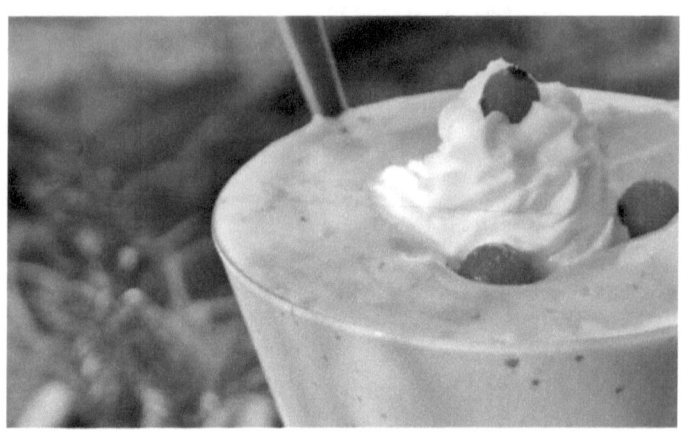

Ingredients:

- 4 medium-sized bananas, cut into 1-inch pieces and frozen
- 1 cup frozen cherries
- 1/2 teaspoon vanilla extract
- 1 tablespoon to 1/4 cup unsweetened almond milk, as needed
- 2 tablespoons mini vegan chocolate chips

Directions:

1. Combine the banana, cherries, and vanilla in a food processor as you add the almond milk one

tablespoon at a time (as needed).
2. Pulse the chocolate chips into the mix.
3. Serve immediately for a soft serve consistency or let sit for a few minutes to achieve a thick milkshake quality. Top with homemade whipped topping and cherries, if desired.

Thick and Creamy Tomato Soup

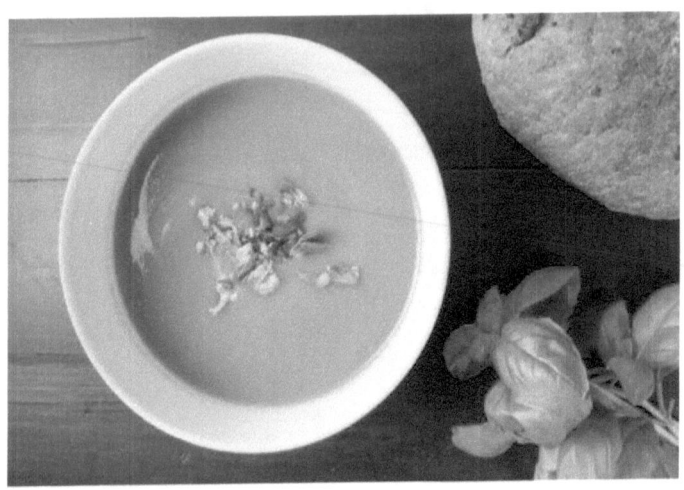

Soup Ingredients:

- 2 tbsp olive oil
- 1 small white onion, peeled and thinly sliced
- 3 cloves garlic, peeled and minced
- 1 (28 oz) can whole peeled tomatoes
- 1/2 cup vegetable stock
- 1/2 cup cashew cream, recipe follows
- 2-3 tsp. granulated sugar
- 1/2 tsp oregano
- 1/4 tsp red pepper flakes, optional
- Salt and pepper, to taste

Kick-start Your Plant-Based Lifestyle

Cashew Cream Ingredients:

- 1/2 cup raw cashews
- 1/4 cup water
- 1 tbsp. fresh lemon juice
- 1/2 tsp. salt

Directions:

1. Combine all the cashew cream ingredients together in a high-powered bender. Place water at the bottom. Blend until smooth and then set aside.
2. In a soup pot, heat two tablespoons of olive oil over medium heat. Add the onions and garlic to make fragrant and translucent (about 5 minutes).
3. Add the tomatoes, vegetable broth, cashew cream, sugar, and spices and beat the mix with the back of a wooden spoon. Bring to a boil and then let simmer for about 10 minutes. Turn off the heat.
4. Pour into blender and blend until smooth. Serve and enjoy!

Kick-start Your Plant-Based Lifestyle

Hey my valued reader, did you enjoy my Summer Recipes? Which one was your favorite so far? Let me know by leaving an Amazon review right now!

I can't wait to hear from you. Thank you!

In The Fall

The fall brings with it gourds and root vegetables of all sorts. Your plant-based diet is sure to be filled with a variety of tastes during this beautiful crisp season!

- Pears: High in flavonoids, antioxidants, and fiber, pears are great for controlling your weight and even fighting diabetes and cardiovascular disease, among others.

- Sweet Potatoes: Iron, calcium, and selenium are just some of the minerals packed into sweet potatoes. This root vegetable boosts the immune system and can even provide joint pain relief.

- Brussel Sprouts: Fiber, vitamins, and minerals are just some of the things these green little sprouts bring to the table. They can reduce your risk of cancer, prevent disease, and lower inflammation.

- Pumpkin: Get a boost of beta carotene that will protect your eyesight while other nutrients in pumpkin boost your immunity and even lower your cancer risk.

Caramelized Pears & Oats

This hearty breakfast treat will get you ready to start your day right.

(no photo for this recipe.)

Ingredients:

- 3/4 cup steel-cut oats
- 1 1/2 cups water
- 1 1/2 Tbsp olive oil
- 2-3 Tbsp brown sugar
- 2 Bosc pears, peeled, cored, and chopped
- 1/4 tsp cinnamon
- 1 Tbsp lemon juice

Directions:

1. Start the oats by boiling water in a small saucepan. Add a pinch of salt and the oats to the boiling water. Swirl and then cover and let cook on low heat for 15 minutes.
2. Prepare the pears by heating a medium saucepan over medium heat. Add the olive oil once hot. After it bubbles, add the brown sugar and stir. Add the pears immediately along with the lemon

juice and cinnamon. Stir to coat. Cover to let steam for about 10 minutes.
3. Remove the lid from the pear pan once they have become tender and golden brown. Let caramelize for a little while over low heat and then remove the pan from the heat.
4. Divide your oats into two bowls and top with the pears. Pecans can also be mixed in for extra flavor and crunch.

Sweet Potato Casserole

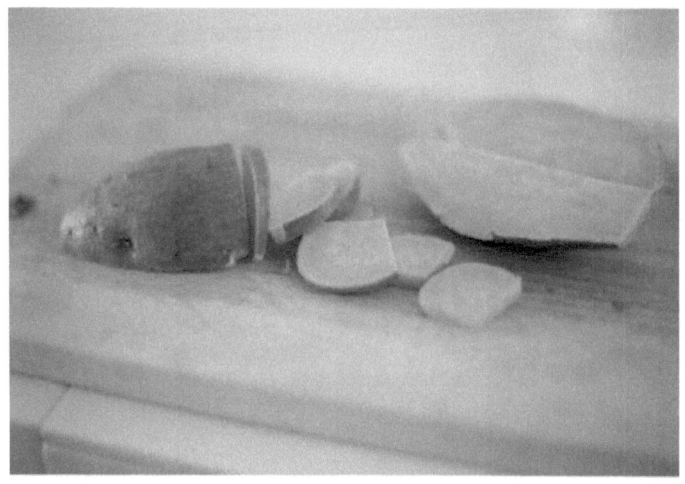

Casserole Ingredients:

- 6 cups cubed sweet potatoes
- 1/2 cup non-dairy milk
- 1/4 cup brown sugar
- 2 tbsp vegan butter
- 1 tsp vanilla extract
- 1 tsp cinnamon
- 1/4 tsp nutmeg
- 1/2 tsp salt

Pecan Topping Ingredients:

- 3/4 cup pecans

Kick-start Your Plant-Based Lifestyle

- 1/3 cup all-purpose flour
- 1/4 cup brown sugar
- 1/2 tsp cinnamon
- 1/4 tsp salt
- 2 tbsp vegan butter, melted

Directions:

1. Preheat your oven to 350 degrees F.
2. Bring 8 cups of water to a boil in a large saucepan. Peel and chop about three large sweet potatoes. Boil for ten minutes, until tender.
3. Prepare the pecan crust by combining everything but the butter in a food processor. Pulse to combine. Add the melted butter as the food processor continues to run. Pulse until fully combined and then set aside.
4. Drain the water from your cooked potatoes and let cool for 10 minutes. Mash and then add the remaining ingredients to the potatoes inside a blender. Blend to combine.
5. Put the sweet potato casserole mix into a dish and then top with the pecan topping. Bake for 20 to 25 minutes until golden brown.
6. Let cool for 10 minutes and then serve.

Maple Balsamic Brussels Sprouts

Brussels sprouts aren't a popular fall vegetable, but they offer plenty of benefits and a lot of flavor when prepared correctly. The glaze in this recipe really adds that extra interest that will have you wanting seconds.

(no photo for this recipe.)

Ingredients:

- 4 cups Brussels sprouts, halved
- 2 tablespoons olive oil
- 1/2 red onion, thinly sliced
- 2-3 garlic cloves, minced
- 1 teaspoon dried rosemary
- salt and pepper, to taste
- 1/3 cup hazelnuts, roasted chopped

Glaze Ingredients:

- 3 tablespoons balsamic vinegar
- 2 teaspoon maple syrup

Directions:

1. Preheat your oven to 425 degrees F.
2. Wash and half your Brussels sprouts. Toss with oil, onions, garlic, rosemary, salt, and pepper. Spread

onto a greased pan and bake for 30 minutes. Let brown and tender before removing from oven and setting aside.
3. Stir the balsamic vinegar and maple syrup together.
4. Remove your sprouts from the oven and toss with hazelnuts. Toss with maple balsamic glaze.
5. Serve warm and enjoy.

Pumpkin Bread

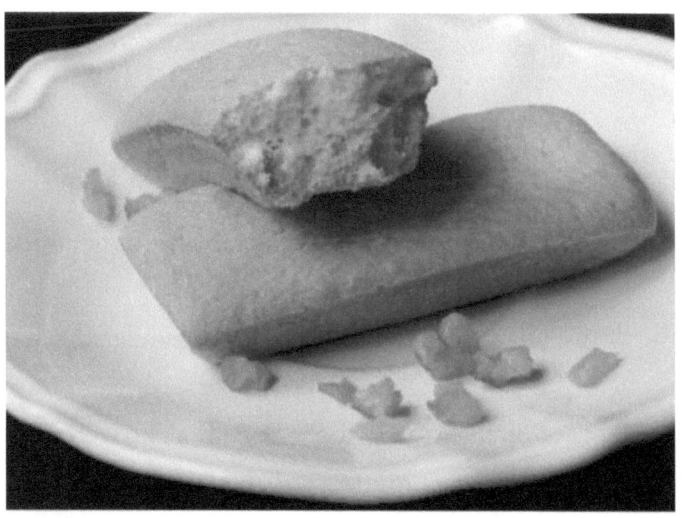

Ingredients:

- 2 cups spelt flour
- 1/2-3/4 cup of coconut, turbinado or organic pure cane sugar
- 1 teaspoon baking powder
- 1 teaspoon baking soda
- 2 heaping teaspoons pumpkin pie spice mix
- pinch of mineral salt
- 1-2 teaspoons vanilla extract
- 1/3 cup water or unsweetened almond milk
- 1/3 cup applesauce

Kick-start Your Plant-Based Lifestyle

- 1 can (15 oz) 100% pumpkin puree
- small handful of pumpkin seeds for topping (optional)

Directions:

1. Preheat your oven to 350 degrees F.
2. Combine the flour, baking powder, baking soda, spices, and salt in a medium bowl.
3. In a small bowl, combine the apple sauce, sugar, water/milk, and vanilla.
4. Add the wet mix to the dry mix along with the pumpkin puree. Mix well, but do not over mix. There should be no clumps. Adjust sweetness to taste.
5. Pour your batter into a greased loaf pan. Bake for 55-60 minutes.
6. Let cool slightly and serve.

In The Winter

The winter season is famous for baking. But, there are all sorts of things that you can do with the delicious seasonal ingredients that accompany the cold weather.

- Pomegranates: Antioxidants and Vitamin C boast cancer prevention properties along with a host of benefits for your immune system. Your digestion will also benefit, making this a famous health food.

- Winter Squash: Manganese and copper are two of the major minerals found in Winter Squash. Butternut and Acorn squash are two of the absolute healthiest.

- Kale: Boost your well-being with antioxidants and a good dose of calcium. Vitamin K and Vitamin C are also found in kale.

- Clementine: Prevent the damage of free radicals, soothe your digestive system, and so much more with this Vitamin C rich fruit. It can even relieve stress and aid weight loss.

Chocolate Pomegranate Fudge Tart

While you can make a delicious pomegranate and spinach salad, sometimes chocolate is the best way to introduce yourself to a new ingredient. So, try this delicious and rich fudge tart to see what pomegranates can offer you.

(no photo for this recipe.)

Crust Ingredients:

- 1 cup pitted dates
- 1 cup walnuts (or nuts of choice)
- pinch of salt

Filling Ingredients:

- 1½ cup cocoa powder or raw cacao
- 1 cup + 2 tablespoons pure maple syrup or honey
- ¾ cup coconut oil, melted
- 1 teaspoon vanilla
- pinch of salt
- ⅛ cup pomegranate arils, plus more for sprinkling on top

Directions:

1. For the crust, place your ingredients into a food processor and blend until finely ground. Pour into

a pan of your choice and firmly press up sides and onto the bottom. Freeze as you prepare the filling.
2. In a large bowl, combine the cocoa powder, maple syrup, coconut oil, vanilla, and salt and whisk. Fold in the pomegranate arils.
3. Pour your filling into the chilled crust. Smooth the top. Sprinkle more rails and place into fridge for 30 minutes until firm.
4. Remove the tart from the pan and cut into slices. Serve at room temperature and store in refrigerator.

Stuffed Acorn Squash

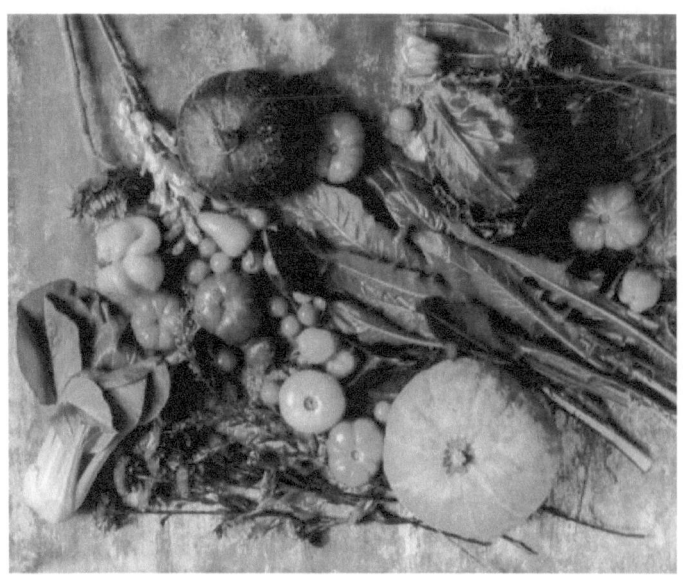

Roasting Ingredients:

- 2 tablespoons of olive oil
- 3 large acorn squash, cut in half and seeds removed
- Salt and pepper

Stuffing Ingredients:

- 1 tablespoon olive oil
- 1 medium onion, chopped
- 3 stalks of celery (¾ cup), chopped

Kick-start Your Plant-Based Lifestyle

- 1 large apple, peeled and cut into small cubes
- 2 cloves of garlic, minced
- 2 1/2 cups cooked quinoa
- ¾ cups dried cranberries
- ½ cup pecans, coarsely chopped
- 1 teaspoon salt
- ½ teaspoon black pepper
- ¼ cup fresh parsley, chopped plus more as garnish

Directions:

1. Preheat the oven to 400 degrees F and line a pan with parchment paper.
2. Drizzle olive oil into the insides of the acorn squash. Use a brush to spread it over the flesh. Sprinkle each half with salt and pepper. Place cut side down onto the pan and roast for 40 minutes, until tender. Let cool for five minutes.
3. Make the stuffing by heating olive oil in a large pan over medium high heat. Add the onion and celery, then cook. Stir frequently for about 5-6 minutes so they become translucent. Add the apply and cook for another 4 minutes until soft. Stir in the garlic and cook for additional 30 seconds.

4. Throw in the quinoa, cranberries, pecans, and salt and pepper. Stir and turn the heat to medium low. Let cook for 8 minutes while stirring. Add some water if it begins to dry out. Adjust seasoning to taste then stir in the parsley.
5. Fill each half with your stuffing and garnish before serving.

Kale Nachos

Bring this to your next party and people will surely give it a curious taste. Anyone who's nervous to try it will quickly become convinced when they are met with its incredible flavor.

(no photo for this recipe.)

Chip Ingredients:

- 1 large bundle curly kale
- 2-3 Tbsp avocado oil or melted coconut oil
- 1 healthy pinch each sea salt + black pepper
- 1 tsp chili powder
- 1 tsp cumin
- 1 Tbsp nutritional yeast

Black Bean Ingredients:

- 1 (15 oz) can of black beans
- 1 tsp ground cumin
- 1 tsp chili powder

Sweet Potato Ingredients:

- 1 Tbsp coconut or avocado oil
- 1 large sweet potato, sliced into 1/4-inch rounds

Toppings:

- Ripe avocado
- Salsa
- Fresh chopped cilantro
- Sliced red onion

Directions:

1. Preheat the oven to 225 degrees F.
2. Add kale to a mixing bowl and drizzle with oil. Disperse it evenly. Add the salt, pepper, chili powder, cumin, and nutritional yeast. Toss to combine.
3. Divide the kale between two large pans. Do not overlap to ensure crispness. Bake each pan for 15 minutes. Toss and then bake for another 5-10 minutes until the kale chips are crispy and slightly brown. Do not burn.
4. Add the partially drained black beans to a small saucepan. Add the cumin and chili powder. Add salt if the beans are not salted. Warm over medium heat. Reduce to low once it simmers. Stir occasionally.
5. Heat a large skillet over medium heat and add a tablespoon of oil to the hot pan. Add sliced sweet

potatoes and cover to steam. Cook for 3-5 minutes. Brown the underside then flip and brown the other side. Cover and continue cooking until brown and tender (about 8 minutes total).
6. Arrange your kale chips on a platter and top with sweet potatoes, black beans, and your desired toppings. Serve as an entree for two or serve four guests with this as a side dish.

Clementine Cupcakes

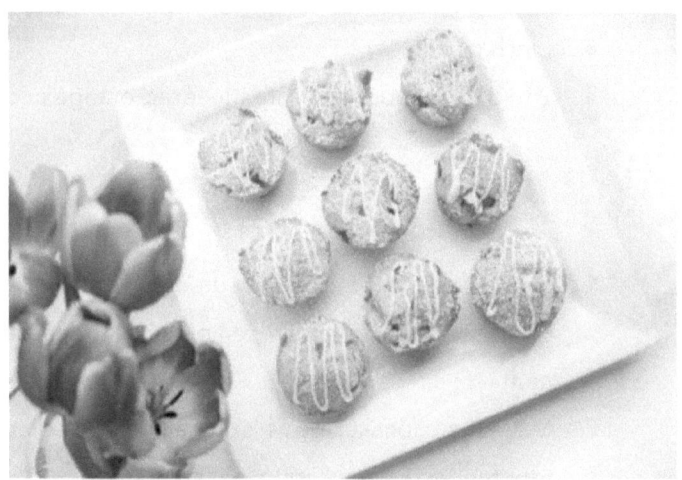

Cupcake Ingredients:

- 2 1/4 cups of all-purpose flour
- 1 cup sugar
- 3/4 teaspoon salt
- 1 teaspoon baking powder
- 1/2 teaspoon baking soda
- 1 cup peeled, diced seedless clementines
- 1 teaspoon vanilla extract
- 1/3 cup vegetable oil
- 1 cup orange juice or tangerine juice

Frosting Ingredients:

- 2 1/4 cups confectioners' sugar, sifted
- pinch of salt
- 2 to 3 tablespoons freshly squeezed orange juice

Directions:

1. Preheat your oven to 400 degrees F. Lightly grease and flour a muffin pan or line with greased muffin tins.
2. Make the cupcakes by whisking all dry ingredients together and then stirring in the chopped clementines.
3. In another bowl, whisk the vanilla, vegetable oil, and orange juice.
4. Stir the wet ingredients into the dry ingredients, but do not over-mix. Spoon the batter into the muffin cups until each is nearly full. Bake for 15 to 18 minutes until domed. They will not brown but you can test for doneness with a toothpick (it should come out clean).
5. Let sit for five minutes and then transfer cupcakes to a wire rack to cool completely.
6. Make the frosting by whisking all ingredients together. Add orange juice little by little until the

right consistency is reached.
7. Frost the cupcakes as you like. Serve and enjoy!

Last Words…

A wise woman once said, "learn five things really well on a topic that you're interested in, and you will become an expert on that topic."

So, well done! You are now officially a plant-based recipes expert.

Not just that, but you are a plant-based recipes expert for any time of the year.

Now how many people could say that about themselves?

Remember to post your photos on Instagram and #PlantBasedDietChallenge!

Kick-start Your Plant-Based Lifestyle

So! How was the book? Did it bring value to you? I sure hope it did, considering you have come to the last page.

Well, reviews are really helpful for small independent writers like me. So it would help me out a lot if you could leave this book an honest review on Amazon.com right now.

I am truly thankful that you have downloaded this book.

Lastly, for more information on health, fitness and wellness, I recommend you check out WorkoutWellnessHub.com and follow their official W.W.H's social media accounts @WorkoutWellnessHub on Facebook and Instagram.

www.ingramcontent.com/pod-product-compliance
Lightning Source LLC
Chambersburg PA
CBHW021813170526
45157CB00007B/2574